Color Star Diet

BY

Paty Rivera

TRANSLATED BY

Claudia Romay

Acknowledgements

First of all, I would like to thank you, Jesus, my God and my teacher, for guiding me in the daily path of discovering that the foods you designed are the best possible fuel to make this wonderful body you gave us work to its highest potential.

I thank my husband Renán for his unconditional love, for being my best friend, and for how fully happy my life has been by his side.

I also want to thank my children Paulina, Andrés, and Mariana, for giving me the ability to love, for always supporting me, and for transmitting me their joy, enthusiasm, and tenacity.

Thanks to my grandson Santiago for teaching me to enjoy every single moment, to my siblings, cherished companions, and to my parents for being an inspiration in my life, as well as for their full and constant dedication.

Contents

Prologue

We live in an accelerated world, one in which we lack the time to take proper care of our health. We need a practical and functional diet that guides us in making healthy choices and improves our quality of life.

By helping you to visualize an adequate food combination, The Color Star Diet will give you the freedom to enjoy all the aspects of your life without having to spend every day counting calories.

Additionally, thanks to The Color Star Diet, you will discover a new way of eating right that will allow you to reach your ideal weight, making you the healthy, dynamic, and productive person you have always wished to be.

By changing the way you eat, you will notice an improvement in both your physical and mental performance: your concentration and memory will sharpen, your percentage of total body fat will diminish, and your muscle mass will increase.

Thanks to this diet, you'll have the chance to lose weight without being hungry. Once free from anxiety and from a compulsion for food, you will be able to maintain optimal hormone levels, which will in turn permit you to burn stored fat.

Furthermore, thanks to The Color Star Diet, you will be able to normalize your blood pressure, cholesterol and triglyceride levels, increase bone calcification, and enforce your immune system, lowering the risk of disease.

In short, by following The Color Star Diet you will improve every aspect of your life, living not only longer, but also better.

How did The Color Star Diet come about?

Nearly twenty years ago, when I finished my degree in Nutrition, I began working in Mexico City's General Hospital, treating overweight and obese patients. It was while attending nutrition clinics that I verified the huge effort people made to lose weight following traditional, low-calorie diets. They were constantly hungry and continuously thinking about what they had to eat. They even reached the point of abandoning their social life because of having to prepare special food for themselves.

Being on a diet caused such suffering that people followed it for some time until they eventually gave up without lacking feelings of impotence and frustration. Most patients ended up not going back to the clinic at all, looking for a magical method that would help them lose weight... sometimes even putting their own health at risk. They would turn to all sorts of diets, some containing a high percentage of animal fats (with the consequent risk of cardiovascular disease), and some others sustained on drugs and pills of unknown origin (which usually tamper with the nervous and circulatory systems).

With time, I came to realize that the diets we worked with did not actually work, and only provoked a profound feeling of guilt on whoever followed them.

One day, after about six months of working at the hospital, I met Cecilia, an encounter that completely changed the course of my life.

Cecilia was an obese woman who was admitted to the hospital by the Endocrinology Department, waiting for the right time to undergo spine surgery.

Two weeks before, she had said goodbye to her husband and children with tears in her eyes. She had put all of her effort into losing weight... and she hadn't been able to do it. Therefore, she now had to be hospitalized for at least a month in order to be strictly subjected to a rigorous diet and hence obtain bigger chances of being able to walk again.

She felt discouraged, for she had been fighting constantly against her fearsome overweight problem since puberty. She had tried all sorts of diets with no result. She even got to the point of taking weight-losing drugs, but her effort still rendered no results. She always regained the lost weight quite quickly. She looked at herself in the mirror and felt depressed, asking herself if she'd ever be able to be thin and healthy like so many people she knew. Yet her dream seemed to drift farther away as time passed.

She had been offered help through rigid diets and pre-established menus provided by doctors. Every time she embarked on a new diet, she got very enthused, bought all that was needed, and prepared all the menus provided, but by the third day hunger attacks and bad moods killed her motivation, which took her back to the doctor both sad and disappointed.

She hated scales, which never failed to denounce her failure and declare her guilty. Her weight began to cause her serious back pain, making it very difficult for her to stand straight. One day, the unbearable pain made her consult an orthopedist, who diagnosed a severe backbone deviation and warned that the only way of obtaining good results after treatment was to lose weight before surgery.

I first met Cecilia in the General Hospital. It was a Thursday. A doctor and I were directing the weekly clinics for weight loss, where all the hospitalized patients came down to an auditorium to receive balanced diet recommendations, recipes, and advice on supporting one another.

Suddenly Cecilia stood up and sobbingly declared she felt terrible and apathetic, hungry and moody, and was beginning to lose the will to live. Her intervention unleashed a reservoir of controversy where patients complained one over the other, stating they were making a huge effort and getting scarce results in return.

I left the auditorium feeling sad and disconcerted, trying very hard, with all the nutrition knowledge available to me, to help these people become healthy and thin... yet I still felt disarmed.

From that day on, I dedicated myself to read and investigate everything related to nutrition, and to taking all the courses my schedule permitted, looking all the time for a diet that would help one get thinner in a healthy manner.

And finally... I found it.

It happened one day while I was taking a specialized course in obesity when, in a book, I ran across a term that would change the course of my life: The "Glycemic Index."

I discovered that in order to lose weight, the secret resided in detecting the velocity with which carbohydrates –or sugars– reached the bloodstream, finding therefore a balance in which the brain can find the fuel it needs to function, and leaving the muscles without any circulating fuel, forcing them to use up fat reserves.

It is thus that I devoted myself to designing a different kind of diet, one that would be aimed mostly towards recovering my patients' health. A diet that promptly permitted me to witness surprising results: some patients have surpassed the goal of losing up to 110 pounds. Today, seeing them thin and healthy makes me feel delighted. Those who had high cholesterol or triglyceride levels have made significant changes in their lives by reducing them considerably, claiming now to have a life full of energy and vitality.

Getting Christmas calls from people who have lost 40 to 45 pounds to thank me and tell me just how radical the change has been in their life is, indeed, a deep satisfaction. One of these people once told me, "I feel like I've bought a ticket to finally live life fully." Another told me, "I thought it was going to be harder, yet I've lost weight seamlessly."

The important thing is that they've learned a healthy way to eat, and have lost several pounds without getting them back.

I hope that in this book you can find a new way to eat without suffering and hunger, as well as without spending all your time counting calories, but rather making a good use of your time enjoying life. And above all, I truly hope all your dreams come true.

I

Diets That Kill

Sometimes, an exasperated need to lose weight leads us to befall upon extremist diets that may severely detriment our health.

Diets High in Fat

Close to 30 years ago, diets high in fat and animal proteins became famous. Dr. Atkins' diet headed the list. This diet allowed unlimited consumption of foods high in saturated fat like sausages, bacon, pork cracklings, eggs, meats, and seafood.

With such a drastic reduction in carb consumption, the body is forced to put a process called ketosis into motion, during which the body produces certain toxic substances called ketone bodies.

Following this kind of diets endangers our health because an excess in saturated fats will cause an increase in cholesterol levels over time, which will, in turn, increase the risk of suffering cardiovascular disease.

Furthermore, excess proteins favors the loss of calcium from our bones, skyrockets uric acid levels, and overloads the kidneys' work.

Any weight loss produced by this diet is related to tissue dehydration: by lacking enough carbs to provide the brain with glucose, the liver's glycogen reserves are utilized, losing three molecules of water per each molecule of glycogen needed.

By eating like this you lose weight quite rapidly, but what you in fact lose is a lot of both muscle mass and water, which is why weight is regained in such a quick manner afterwards.

Fasting Diets

Starvation diets, or diets that require any kind of fasting, make the body interpret the lack of food as a food shortage. Organs reduce their activity in order to save on energy required for life itself, and muscles are consumed. By following this type of diet you lose weight by destroying a good part of your muscles, making it easier to regain weight.

Every kilogram of muscle in the body consumes 46 calories a day, while a kilogram of fat consumes only two. By destroying muscle, fewer calories will be burned per day and fat will end up being stored.

In 1945, thirty people voluntarily accepted to participate in a study about partial fasting in the University of Minnesota. Results were evaluated after 23 weeks of closely following the diet. These people's hair was thin and dull, and their skin was less elastic, just like in old people.

It has also been proven that hypothyroidism can be provoked when subjecting our body to stress while following low calorie diets. When a person doesn't eat enough, his or her metabolism slows, causing feelings of tiredness and sleepiness. When, on the other hand, we go back to our normal eating habits and increase the amount of food we eat, lost weight is quickly regained or even surpassed, because the body is now used to consuming less energy.

These facts are proven by follow-up studies done in prisoners from World War II. Prisoners in concentration camps survived with mere pieces of bread, potatoes, broth and water. When abandoning prison and retaking normal eating habits, their bodies, which had been subject to a high degree of metabolic stress, took advantage of the newly taken food to accumulate as much energy reserves as possible in case a similar situation presented itself.

Anorexia nervosa is one of the most frequent eating disorders seen in our society today. People who suffer it subject themselves to extended fasting periods and begin to consume themselves, destroying their own muscles to satisfy the brain's needs.

Muscle is lost daily on an attempt to survive, because the less muscle there is, the less energy their body consumes. It is like this that the body reduces its energy consumption to its minimum, to the point of having the person survive with a minimum amount of calories until, finally, the heart (which is a muscle as well) begins to be consumed and death finally strikes, in the guise of a cardiovascular problem.

Frequently, this kind of disease presents itself in adolescent girls who, pressured by their peers or by the prototype of today's beautiful women, strive to have a thin body at all costs, driven by this obsession even to the point of flirting with death.

Vegetarian Diets

Studies done on children strictly subject to exclusive vegetarian diets have proven a deficiency of Vitamin B12 and a lack of development of the nervous system.

Human beings can't synthesize a protein component called tryptophan, which is absolutely necessary for the formation of neurons in the brain. Owed to a more complex digestive system in some animals, both cattle and chickens are able synthesize it, and in turn transfer it to eggs, milk and beef, which is why lacto-ovo-vegetarians don't present a deficiency of this amino acid.

If you decide to follow a vegetarian regime, monitor your diet closely. In order to prevent protein, vitamin, and/or mineral deficiencies, make sure you include in your diet a good variety of foods like cheese, egg, soy, spirulina algae, and other leguminous plants and seeds.

High Carb Diets

It was by 1930 that the calorie theory first appeared, and balanced diets began to be designed based on the following equation:

$$Energy\ Intake = Energy\ Output$$

Therefore, if we ingest more calories than those we use up, we end up gaining weight, and if we use up more calories than those we ingest, we're supposed to lose weight.

Based in this theory, the United States Department of Agriculture (USDA) designed and recommended the Nutritional Pyramid in 1992. They concluded that if carbs provided 4 kilocalories per gram and fats provided 9, we would lose weight and improve our health by increasing the consumption of carb-rich cereals and lowering that of oils or fats.

Hence, the food pyramid recommends the consumption of 6 to 11 rations of cereal a day with a minimum of fats.

As the recommendations of the food pyramid took force, light products appeared, low in fat but rich in carbs. Ice creams and yogurts rich in cornstarch, as well as granola bars, biscuits, and cookies rich in sugars and carbs emerged... but, oh yeah! Low in fat. Even some light cheeses that had been rid of fat got cornstarch or mashed potatoes added.

After years of following this kind of diet, statistical research was done with surprising results: the amount of overweight people almost doubled in 12 years. By 1988, 35% of women were overweight, while by the year 2000 the percentage surpassed 52.5%.

According to Mexico's National Institute of Statistics and Geography (*INEGI* by its acronym in Spanish), 16.4% of Mexican women were overweight by 1988. In 1999, the number had gone up to 30%.

Statistics in the US have been no less alarming: according to data reported by CNN's Harris Poll of May, 2002, obesity is escalating to epidemic proportions. Eighty percent of Americans over 25 years old is overweight, and obesity percentages in children have doubled.

Diabetes Type II, which normally appears during adulthood, was another disease that alarmingly increased in incidence as a result of the so-called light diet. This disease presents itself in obese people who live a sedimentary life and follow a carb-rich diet (sugars, flours, candies, sodas, and desserts).

In fact, if concrete measures aren't taken in order to prevent it, diabetes may become the first cause of death over the next few years. Ten years ago, diabetes was the fifth mortality cause; today it reigns in third.

Why has the number of diabetes patients increased?

When people abuse carb consumption by basing their diet in cereals and sodas, blood sugar levels increase abruptly, favoring insulin production. Insulin is a hormone produced by the pancreas to permit the passage of glucose into our cells.

Those cells that don't need so much sugar start to become resistant to insulin and, with the years, the pancreas gets tired of working excessively until it stops producing insulin. And that's when diabetes kicks in.

The kidneys begin to get rid of excess sugar, increasing the need to urinate and causing intense thirst and appetite. Vision becomes blurry and people feel tired and sleepy.

If not treated on time, diabetes can cause serious complications like blindness, renal insufficiency, arteriosclerosis, and heart attack.

Diabetes has become an epidemic in times in which we are incited to eat and eat and keep eating cereals and refined sugars that progressively damage the pancreas until it stops working.

Hypertriglyceridemia (an increase in blood's triglycerides levels), a disease also related to an excess of carbs in the blood, has been related to a higher rate in heart attacks.

When informed of having high levels of blood triglycerides, people tend to relate it with fat consumption and begin to take fat out of their diets. Nevertheless, the blood's triglyceride level is directly related to carb consumption.

If we eat cereals or refined sugars in large amounts, blood sugar levels skyrocket and we end up storing them as triglycerides or fat. Sometimes, these substances return to the blood and elevate the levels of blood triglycerides.

After analyzing several kinds of diets, we have become aware of the risks involved in following those diets that dangle from extremes.

It is by learning to eat in a balanced way that we will be able to obtain both health and life..

II

The Secret for Weight Loss

After evaluating the results high-carb diets throw, we may feel disconcerted.

If carbs provide 4 kilocalories, while fats provide 9, how is it that people get fatter even while eating less fat? The answer lies in the fact that in order to get thinner, counting calories alone does not do the trick. Above all, what really helps is to provide fuel only to the brain while maintaining blood sugar levels stable.

How much you eat is not the only thing that is important, but *what* you eat as well: 100 calories from a baked potato are not the same as 100 calories from cheese or cantaloupe. This is because the production of insulin (the storage hormone), depends greatly on the type of food consumed.

What is Insulin?

Insulin is a hormone produced by the pancreas whose function is to allow the passage of sugars from the blood into the liver and into muscle cells, as well as to store any leftover sugar as fat.

Insulin production is stimulated when eating carbs that raise blood sugar levels. When eating them in excess, leftover sugar in the blood ends up stored as fat.

Where Can We Find These Sugars or Carbohydrates?

Most of us know that carbs can be found in sodas, pastries, cookies, sugar and honey. Nevertheless, savory foods (like rice, bagels, potatoes, and tortillas) also contain sugars or carbs.

In fact, carbs can be found in a great variety of foods such as cereals, fruits, milk, yogurt, legumes, and some vegetables.

Most people who wish to lose weight begin their day with a breakfast based on fruit, milk, and cereal. Soon you can hear them saying, "Even without eating any fat, I can't lose weight."

What Happens When We Eat a Lot of Carbs in One Meal?

To understand the function of carbs in our body, let's imagine that a slice of bread is similar to a train made up of several cars, each loaded with sugar, which comes in through our mouth. When they come in contact with saliva, the train cars begin to separate with the help of ptyalin (a salivary enzyme, also known as salivary amylase, that begins the digestion of carbs), after which they pass into the esophagus, the stomach and, finally, into the small intestine, where they are absorbed and taken into the blood.

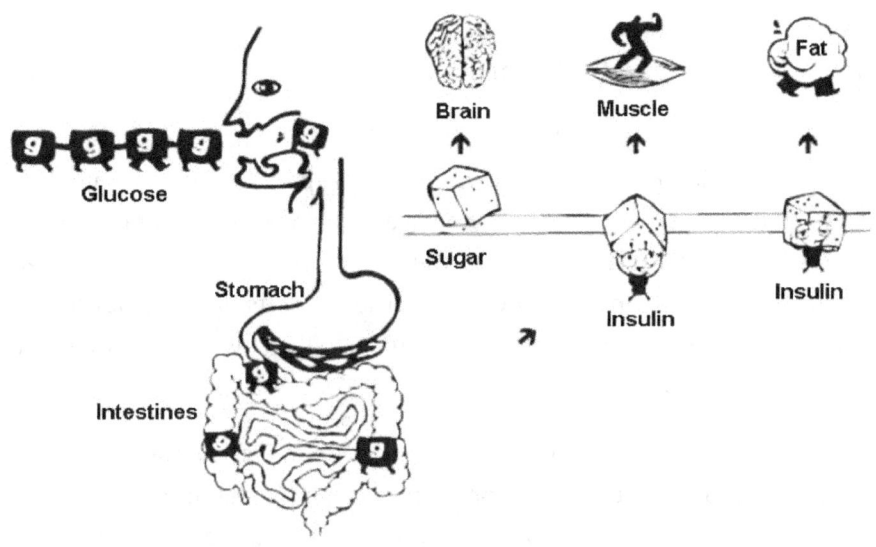

Once in the blood, the train cars unload their sugar content, elevating blood sugar levels.

The brain needs sugar, or glucose, to function correctly. Since our body's priority is the brain's health, the brain is the only one that can take sugar directly from the blood, without needing help from insulin.

If the brain detects that there is still sugar in the blood after it has taken the amount of sugar it needs, it signals the pancreas to secrete the hormone insulin, which when reaching the blood allows the passage of sugar into the liver and into muscle cells. Once our liver and muscles have all the sugar they need, excess sugar is deposited as fat in adipose tissue

Therefore, a diet high in carbs increases insulin production and ends up converting excess sugars into fat. But this is not the worst part, though, for once sugar is stored, blood sugar levels drop below normal and provoke a hypoglycemic state.

Two or three hours later, the brain needs sugar again and cannot find it. Mental agility decreases and people begin to feel bad tempered, sleepy and without concentration, in addition to getting a crave for whatever they can get their hands on.

Eating high quantities of carbs, therefore, makes us fall into a vicious circle in which eating pushes us to keep eating. On one hand, we raise blood sugar levels above what can be expected (hyperglycemia), increasing insulin production. On the other, insulin allows the passage of sugars into cells and ends up storing them as fats, making blood sugar levels descend and creating a state of hypoglycemia, which makes us crave sweet food.

High-carb diets, like the one recommended by the Nutritional Pyramid, create a sugar addiction along a huge feeling of frustration and guilt. It asks us to eat from 1,000 to 1,200 calories, but they also recommend so many carbs that we feel a crazy need of eating again and again. Little by little, we become enslaved by carbs and end up believing those extra pounds are our fault, because of our weak will.

A few months ago, a marathon runner came into my office. He told me he felt tired and sleepy, that his energy levels had collapsed, and he could not understand why.

When questioning him about his eating habits I immediately identified his problem: a high-carb diet. For breakfast he had orange juice and a biscuit with jam. Sometimes, he added a serving of fresh fruit with granola and honey.

At midmorning he ate some oat cookies with a sports beverage.

By lunchtime, he was starving. He then ate a plate of pasta with roasted vegetables, a baked potato and a stew, along with sugar-sweetened fruit juice.

By nighttime, cookies and milk, fruit and yogurt were in order. I explained to him that he had become a carb victim, and that, with his daily diet, he was causing himself hypoglycemia (a decline in sugar levels). That's why he felt so tired.

By limiting his carbs and increasing his protein and polyunsaturated fat consumption, his life changed and his energy levels increased, as did his physical and mental performance.

What Is The Secret?

The secret for reaching your ideal weight, improving your health, and increasing your energy levels resides in controlling insulin production while maintaining blood sugar levels stable.

On one hand, when blood sugar levels descend below normal, we feel weak and irritable, losing our concentration and becoming less productive. On the other hand, when these levels rise above normal, insulin is produced and fat is stored in adipose tissue, causing an overweight or obesity problem.

CARB EXCESS = HYPERINSULINISM + OBESITY

Since 1979, nutrition scientists have proved through research that a metabolic process for weight gain exists, reaching the conclusion that hyperinsulinism is present in all cases of obesity in a proportional way to the magnitude of obesity.

This means that if you're only 10 or 20 pounds above your ideal weight, you suffer of moderate hyperinsulinism, while if you are 70 to 80 pounds above, your hyperinsulinism is severe.

This leads us to the following conclusion: one of the differences between a thin person and an obese one is that the first produces less insulin than the second.

A very worrying fact is that 7 out of every 10 people is overweight, a state which, in itself, is a risk factor for diabetes, hypertension, arthritis, hyperlipidemia, and depression. Three hundred thousand deaths a year are related to obesity.

The risk of suffering a heart attack, angina, embolism, and cerebral infarctions is two to three times greater in obese people.

What can we do to produce less insulin and prevent being overweight or obese? Some studies made on diabetic patients reveal surprising results based in food's Glycemic Index.

Testimonies

Incredible, but true. If ever there was something I didn't believe in, it was nutriology. For over 30 years, I had tried to lose weight with all kinds of doctors: iridologists, bariatricians, homeopaths, even charlatans. And, oh! The roads I had traveled in my desire to lose weight... what was vanity at first later became a necessity.

I am 46 years old, have a young child, and was beginning to have serious health problems. The doctor had prescribed a blood pressure pill, and when asking him how long I had to take it, he said, "Until you lose weight." A year went by, and I was still fighting my weight. Until one day, someone recommended me to see Paty Rivera, the nutriologist. The first time I went to see her, I was in a terrible condition: there were 128 pounds of excess fat in my body.

She recommended me to stop eating sugars and refined flours, and actually gave me the magic recipe when she said,

"You're eating too many carbohydrates. That is why you're always hungry and anxious to eat sweets and foods prepared with flours."

Paty taught me how to eat through the Color Star Diet and, thanks to God, to her help, and to my force of will, I've lost 123 pounds. I'm not done yet... but this is the final sprint. My life has completely changed, and the doctor has allowed me to stop taking the blood pressure pill. I now am an agile, healthy, happy person.

S. Garza

III

Food's Glycemic Index

One of the latest discoveries in the nutrition field is that insulin production depends not only on the amount of sugars that reach the blood, but also on the speed with which these carbs are digested and absorbed.

Such velocities are measured with food's **Glycemic Index**.

Thanks to the discovery of food's Glycemic Index we are able to lose weight and improve our health.

The Glycemic Index is measured in foods containing sugars or carbs that, when digested and absorbed through the intestine, increase blood sugar levels.

The speed with which these sugars or carbs are absorbed depends on the type of nutrients they contain, the amount of fiber present, and the composition of any other foods present in the stomach and intestine during digestion.

Foods containing sugars that reach the blood at high speed are known as *High Glycemic Index Foods*. Foods whose sugars reach the blood slowly are known as *Low Glycemic Index Foods*.

Problems Caused by Foods with a High Glycemic Index

When eating any food with a High Glycemic Index, its sugars are absorbed rapidly, which abruptly increases blood sugar levels. The brain uptakes the amount of sugar it needs to work well, but then detects more sugar in the blood than it needs. As a result, it sends a signal to the pancreas to have it produce insulin in great amounts. Insulin acts as a gatekeeper, allowing the passage of sugars into cells. If muscle cells are not able to burn all those sugars, the excess is stored as fat in adipose tissue.

The higher the Glycemic Index of a food, the greater the amount of insulin produced by the body. This is why *carb-containing* foods don't always cause the same amount of insulin to be produced in the body.

Some foods are better than others, depending on the type of nutrients they contain.

Fruits and raw vegetables contain considerable quantities of fiber, which decreases the absorption speed of sugars in the intestine. In contrast, the sugars in white bread and in potatoes are absorbed at great speed, favoring the production of insulin, the expert in storing fat.

To measure a food's Glycemic Index, a glucose solution was given to a group of volunteers. Since glucose is the blood's sugar, it was given a value of 100% in its absorption speed.

Afterwards, the absorption speeds of different foods were registered and then compared with the glucose's speed. Sugars in most fruits reached the blood slowly, in a speed 40% to 50% that of glucose, while sugars from cereals made it in 80% to 90%.

These results were startling for some scientists. Before discovering the Glycemic Index, it was thought that sugars from fruits were digested faster than complex carbs found in cereals.

Now we know the opposite is true. Most fruits have a Low Glycemic Index, while cereals have a High one.

A baked potato got a Glycemic Index (GI) of 121, rising above the speed of glucose, while an apple registered a GI of 46.

To understand the importance the Glycemic Index has, let us remember the train example. In the case of cereals, the sugar trains reach the blood at the same time and unload their content, causing an abrupt rise in blood glucose levels and favoring insulin production. In contrast, sugars from fruits are digested slowly and reach the blood gradually, without changing blood sugar levels abruptly.

To prevent an insulin overproduction, and therefore the storing of sugars as fat, it is important to reduce the speed with which sugars reach the blood.

Some food's fiber content slows the absorption speed of sugars in the intestine, which is why it is always better to consume whole fruit rather than drinking fruit juice.

Carbs from wild rice reach the blood slowly, while carbs from white rice do it quite rapidly.

Another factor that slows the absorption velocity is the types of nutrients foods have.

Proteins and fats slow carb absorption. Rice, for example, reaches the blood faster than beans, which are rich in protein and fiber.

Cereals, not requiring digestion in the stomach, pass directly into the intestine and are absorbed immediately. Proteins, on the other hand, need the stomach's chlorhydric acid to be digested and thus slow the digestion of whatever else is accompanying them.

Sugars from spaghetti are slow because of their semolina content (a type of protein), while instant soups are quicker because of their high starch content.

In order to slow bread's absorption speed, we can combine it with some cheese or tuna.

Fats also slow the velocity of the stomach's emptying. The first thing to go through the stomach is carbs, followed by proteins and, finally, fats. Since the stomach is constantly moving, any fats we eat get mixed up with the rest of the food, slowing the general absorption speed.

When eating rice with vegetables, we feel full quite fast but then feel hungry in a short period of time. In contrast, if we eat rice, meat and avocado, we feel full longer.

To prevent insulin overproduction the following is recommended: when eating a slice of bread, add some cheese and avocado or a little peanut butter.

The concept of eating right has dramatically changed by discovering about the Glycemic Index. Now we know that eating a baked potato increases our insulin levels more than eating white sugar.

The way foods are prepared also affects sugars' absorption speeds. A raw carrot has a Glycemic Index of 35, while a cooked one increases its GI to 85, owed to a breaking of starches due to heat.

The more we consume raw fruits and vegetables, the more fiber we will have to maintain blood sugar levels stable, which reduces appetite and helps us lose fat.

Insulin Producing Foods	
(High Production) High Glycemic Index	(Low Production) Low Glycemic Index

Glucose	Beans
Baked potato	Lentils
French-Fries	Peas
Mashed Potatoes	Long grain rice
Short grain rice	Pre cooked rice
Instant rice	Whole grain oatmeal
Instant oatmeal	Tomato juice
Instant hot chocolate	Rye bread
White bread	Whole bread
Bread roll or baguette	Raw vegetables
Boiled sweet potato	Raw carrots
Beets	Fresh fruit
Corn Flakes	Spaghetti *al dente*
Banana	Cantaloupe
Mango	Grapefruit

Factors That Lower Sugar's Absorption Speeds

The fiber in some foods slows the absorption of sugars by the intestine. This is why eating raw vegetables like celery, watercress, Swiss chards, spinach, and lettuce, among others, is recommended, just like eating unpeeled fruit. Preferably, fruit juices must be evaded because they take sugar to the blood faster.

Eating some proteins and fats every time a carb is consumed is also recommended because both proteins and fats slow the speed in which sugars reach the blood.

Which Carb Sources are Recommended?

The best is always to choose foods which have carbs with a Low Glycemic Index: yogurt, milk, soy beans, peas, beans, lentils, peaches, apples, plums, pears, cantaloupes, and grapefruits.

Which Carb Sources Are To Be Avoided?

Refined cereals, instant pasta, fruits in syrup, fruit juices, white bread, cooked carrots, bananas, potatoes, popcorn, cookies, pastries, refined-flour tortillas, corn, caramels, sodas, and cookies.

Glycemic Index of some foods			
High Glycemic Index (Bad carbs)		Low Glycemic Index (Good carbs)	
Glucose	100	Wild rice	50
Baked Potato	121	Peas	50
Mashed potatoes	90	Peanuts	21
Honey	90	Whole rice bread	40
Refined sugar	75	Yogurt or milk	35
Chocolate bar	69	Dark chocolate	22
Jams and marmalades	70	Fresh fruit	30
Whole wheat bread	75	Lentils	30
Pasta	78	Soy	20

Doughnuts or waffles	109	Mixed grain bread	48
Processed cereal with sugar	106	Oatmeal	40

Curious Facts

Before food's Glycemic Index was discovered, scientists thought that simple sugars (like refined sugar) were digested quite quickly by the body, increasing the blood's sugar levels, and that complex sugars (like those in cereals) were digested more slowly. Nowadays, we know that simple carbs reach the blood more slowly than complex carbs do. And so, the following approaches were established with which you can improve your eating habits:

- It's better to eat plain sugar than a baked potato
- It's better to eat beans than rice
- If you are going to eat a slice of bread, it's better to combine it with ham or cheese
- A banana that is still ripening is better than a ripe banana, because the latter has more sugars
- It's better to eat powdered fructose that fructose syrup
- White sugar has a lower Glycemic Index than honey
- 14 french-fries increase your insulin level more than a cup of plain sugar

Thus, the Glycemic Index helps us in discovering that losing weight depends not only on counting calories, but also on a hormonal system that is put to work every time we eat.

When sugars reach the blood slowly and little by little, glucose levels are kept stable for up to five hours. This helps us feel full and provides a larger physical and mental energy.

Your health, performance, and productivity will improve as you learn to   choose   carbs   with   Low   Glycemic   Index   for   your   diet

Testimonies

Hello! First of all, let me sincerely congratulate you, Paty, for this wonderfully written book.

If it seems to have vanished from bookstores, it is because I bought a lot of them to give as Christmas presents and because I have recommended it to whomever I could think of.

I bought the book in November, on the 18th to be exact. I liked it so much, I finished it within a day. I had already heard some things about the glycemic index, and with this book I could understand it better.

I started the diet immediately after finishing the book. I had tried starting a "diet" several times last year, but nothing seemed to work. I got discouraged and ate again in an undisciplined manner.

Even so, though, with this book, it was much easier and, for the first time, I finally understood how important our diet is for our health, as well as how we can harm our body without knowing what we are actually doing.

I started the "diet" (since for me this book teaches a healthy eating habit, more than a diet) weighing 155 pounds, and I am 5' 3". As you can see, I was considerably overweight. Nowadays, 3 months later, I've lost 25 pounds effortlessly. With discipline, of course, and with an intense 1-hour walk every morning. I feel amazingly well. I just turned 40 and thanks to this book, I did it honorably.

My children are experts now when it comes to glycemic index and are more conscious of what they eat.

Congratulations... and if I can help promote you, count me in, along with my 25 pounds lost.

Greetings,

Ingrid

IV

The Magical World of Food

We very much worry about material possessions and take good care of them to make them last longer. If we buy a car we provide it with the best possible fuel and tune it up every six months.

As far as we're concerned, natural food is the best possible fuel we can find to have our body function to its maximum capacity.

In order to understand the role food plays in our health, we have classified it by colors, dividing it into four groups.

1. Reds: Proteins

Among them, we can find meat, eggs, chicken, dairy, fish, and seafood. These foods provide us with proteins, calcium, iron, and vitamin D.

Proteins are to us what cement, sand, and wood are to a house.

Proteins are the basic structure of all cells, taking part in blood's hemoglobin and in the genetic code that determines our inherited traits. They play a basic role in the formation of our muscles, bones, hair, skin, and nails. They also intervene in hormone, antibody, and neurotransmitter formation.

Some foods of animal origin contain saturated fats. Therefore, it is important to learn how to choose healthy, low fat protein foods:

- Choose fish over red meats
- When buying meat, choose lean cuts like steak or filet, avoiding chops, ribs, T-bones, or rib eyes.
- Skin both chicken and turkey
- Prefer low fat cheeses, like cottage, skim ricotta or low fat cream cheese, avoiding the likes of Swiss and cheddar cheeses
- Eat three to four eggs a week

Recent research reveals the importance of a high-protein diet. More than 80 thousand nurses participated in a study that lasted 20 years and which showed, in that time, that whoever consumed more proteins presented 75% risk of developing heart disease, whereas those who ate fewer proteins showed a heart disease risk of 100%.

It is believed that those who consumed more protein reduced the consumption of carbs and fats as well.

Excess carb consumption increases triglyceride levels in the blood, in the same way that eating excessive amounts of saturated fat increases circulating cholesterol levels.

In contrast, a good consumption of proteins can help you reach your ideal weight and improve your health. An excess in protein consumption produces uric acid and urea, which may damage the liver and kidneys and cause osteoporosis. Moderation is the key.

Many of my patients have told me about how they got their muscular tone back and reduced their appetite when eating the right amount of reds.

It has been proved that certain amino acids found in protein-rich foods act as appetite suppressors:

- The amino acid L-phenylalanine increases cholecystokinin production, a substance that sends signals to the brain to make us stop eating.
- Another amino acid, tryptophan, increases serotonin production, which decreases the desire to continue eating carbs.
- Six volunteers ingested phenylalanine, which resulted in a 500-calorie reduction through food in their diet.

Proteins stimulate the production of glucagon, a hormone that releases the liver's stored glycogen into the blood, and stabilizes sugar levels, lowering the eagerness to eat.

Snacking with a bit of fresh cheese right before a meal, or beginning a meal with the main course (chicken, meat, or fish) can help you lose weight.

Animal food products also contain **calcium**, specially cheese and some fish and sardines. Ninety-five percent of our body's calcium is deposited in bones, while the other 5% circulates in the blood and is necessary for contracting our muscles.

During menopause, estrogen production fails, lowering calcium absorption in women. Since we require certain percentage of blood calcium for our muscles to contract and for the heart to keep beating, the body begins to use the bone's calcium deposit. With time, bones turn porous and weak, breaking easily. A calcium deficiency causes osteoporosis, the most frequent handicap cause in adults.

The prevention of osteoporosis is not the only important reason for calcium consumption. A new study suggests that calcium also helps prevent hypertension, a silent disease that affects 6.3 million people in the United States.

James H. Dwyer and his colleagues from The University of Southern California (USC) School of Medicine studied 6,634 men and women for a period of 14 years. Results revealed that people who consume at least 1 gram of calcium a day reduced the risk of suffering hypertension by 12%.

Consuming calcium also helps in protecting us against environmental pollution. Calcium is the natural antagonist of lead, protecting us against lead absorption in the intestine when present. Beginning a day with a cheese sandwich or cottage cheese may prevent the risk of lead poisoning.

Foods of animal origin are also rich in vitamin D, which must be consumed for calcium to be absorbed adequately. This vitamin helps make bones and teeth stronger. It is primarily found in cheeses, egg yolks, and some fish.

Sunlight on the skin helps produce vitamin D. This is why sunbaths are recommended for babies and old people, as well as doing activities outside to help our body produce vitamin D and increase calcium absorption.

Recent studies reveal that the incidence of osteoporosis has increased, especially among women who work in artificially illuminated spaces.

Another important ingredient provided by animal foods is iron. It is primarily found in egg yolks and red meat. Iron is a very important mineral that intervenes in the formation of hemoglobin and improves oxygenation in the blood. When people suffer an iron deficiency (called anemia) they feel lethargic and tired, and their skin turns pallid.

In Mexico, anemia is pretty common, especially in children. To lower this deficiency, the government has fortified some foods with iron: boxed cereals, cookies, and some sweet snacks like Twinkies or cupcakes, for example.

Nevertheless, excess iron can also be harmful. The epidemiologist Jukka Salonen and his colleagues in Kuopio University observed 1900 Finnish males between the ages of 42 and 60 for a period of five years, measuring the iron reserves in the body and interrogating them about their diet. During the investigation, 83 patients suffered heart attacks.

Among those with more iron reserves, the risk of suffering a heart attack was twice as high as that of those with less iron.

Walter Willet and colleagues found out that excess iron ingestion increases the risk of suffering coronary insufficiency and heart attacks.

Experts recommend a reduction in red meat consumption, taking vitamin and mineral complements (with no iron added) and cereals that are not fortified with this mineral, as well as donating blood. In a study conducted in Italy, blood donors between the ages of 65 and 69 presented a mortality rate of 50% in contrast to non-donors of the same age.

By 1930, a man who worked in the morgue observed that more men died of heart attacks than women did. Nonetheless, he realized that the number of post-menopausal women or women with hysterectomies who died of heart attacks equaled that of men. This made him think that, somehow, menstruation protected women from suffering a heart attack.

Fifteen years ago, this theory was proved to be somewhat correct. During menstruation, women get rid of iron, a basic blood component. Excess iron in the blood converts to a substance called ferritin, which favors fat oxidation in arteries, causing fat plaques to harden and increasing the risk of a heart attack.

This is why men over 35 and women after menopause or with no uterus must not take multivitamin complexes with iron, as well as prevent eating foods enriched with this mineral.

2. Greens: Vegetables. Free to Eat Whenever You Like

Vegetables are very important for our health, for they provide vitamins, minerals, water, and fiber.

Water is vital. It hydrates us and allows nutrients to be transported to all of our cells.

Vegetables are also a source of fiber, especially when eaten raw or in a salad. Fiber plays a very important role in favoring the health of the digestive system.

Since the human digestive system is incapable of digesting fiber or cellulose, it was thought until recently that fiber had no use, and thus all foods began to be refined. This caused a substitution of fruit consumption by bottled juice, and products made with white sugar and refined flour began to appear in the market.

Years later, while evaluating health statistics in different continents, it was observed that cardiovascular and digestive diseases in Africa were much less. When observing eating habits, Africans were found to be big fiber consumers. They ate whole fruits, vegetables, and integral cereals, while Americans consumed bottled sodas and refined cereals.

Without the necessary fiber, the organism cannot easily eliminate residues and survive illnesses. In contrast, when eating a good salad, fiber acts like a little brush, cleaning the insides of our digestive system.

To understand the function of fiber, we could compare it to a sponge, which when entering the mouth and going down the esophagus, stomach, and intestine, absorbs different liquids (like saliva and digestive juices) and swells, making us feel full. When the intestine's cells detect it as full, peristaltic movements are favored to prepare us for intestinal evacuation.

Imagine a toothpaste container: when full, barely is it pressed and toothpaste comes out easily. The same thing happens with our intestine. When it is empty because of a lack of fiber, food stops and ferments, causing gases and intestinal inflammation.

Raw vegetables also help us get rid of toxins, not only because they are important sources of fiber, but also because the contain enzymes and chlorophyll. Enzymes are substances that the cell requires in order to metabolize carbs, proteins, and fats. They help with cellular respiration and muscle contraction, facilitate digestion and absorptions of nutrients, as well as urine excretion. Chlorophyll enriches blood and helps combat tumor growth, especially in the lungs. It also helps destroy artery clots and lessen the production of lymphatic nodes. Most plants contain chlorophyll, but most especially those that are dark green in color like watercress, Swiss chards, spinach, or broccoli.

Therefore, it is essential to eat 3 cups of raw salad a day, making yours one of the best habits to maintain your good health.

Phytonutrients

According to research made in Cornell University, more than 3,000 phytonutrients have been found in fruits and vegetables. Phytonutrients are substances capable of protecting us against ailments like cancer and cardiovascular disease.

- Sulforaphane, present in broccoli and cauliflower, inhibits the production of cancer cells.
- Allicin, found in garlic, prevents blood clot formation.
- Capsaicin, component of hot chili peppers, blocks attacks made by carcinogenic substances, protecting our cell's DNA.
- Genistein from bean sprouts stops tumor growth.
- Lycopene from tomatoes and lutein from spinach both prevent damage to cells.

Doctor David Heber, founder and director of UCLA's Human Nutrition Center and author of the book *What color is your diet?*, suggests that we eat 5 servings of fruit and vegetables a day, each of different color. Experts are convinced that pigments, which give foods their color, contain phytonutrients capable of preventing disease.

The red color in tomatoes provides lycopene, ideal to prevent prostate cancer, while broccoli's green color contains sulforaphane, which protects against breast cancer.

The blue in eggplants protects the brain and prevents urinary infections, while the orange in pumpkin blossoms promotes better heart health.

"Choose bright food in bright and appetizing colors," recommends Doctor Daniel Nadeau, professor of Tuff Medical School and coauthor of *The Color Code: A Revolutionary Eating Plan for Optimum Health*.

A study made by the Harvard Public Health School revealed that men who consumed foods prepared with tomato ten times a week, had half the incidence of prostate cancer than those who just consumed these foods once a week.

Lycopene, a carotenoid found in tomatoes, is not only associated with fewer incidence of prostate cancer, but is a powerful antioxidant that has been proved to have a protecting effect against both stomach and esophagus cancer.

Eating a good quantity of lycopene every day is not that hard: 2 oz of tomato purée (56 grams) contain more than 23 milligrams of absorbable lycopene. This much lycopene a day provides an optimal level of protection. In truth, raw tomato juice is a poor lycopene source because absorption is very limited in this form. Preparing or cooking tomato with some kind of fat, like olive oil or another vegetable oil, liberates lycopene from inside the tomato's cells, and allows it to effectively cross the intestine's wall and reach our blood stream.

Preparing foods based on cooked tomato, like spaghetti with tomato sauce and olive oil, is recommended.

Beta carotene is another phytonutrient found in dark green colored vegetables like Swiss chards, watercress, and spinach. This ingredient acts like a Vitamin A precursor, favoring good vision. A deficiency in this vitamin provokes night blindness, which prevents us from distinguishing between lights and shadows.

Dark green vegetables are also rich in different kinds of Vitamin B, which are in charge of turning food into energy, and are essential for the nervous system.

Our body does not distinguish between physical and emotional stress. If a rabid dog appeared before us while walking, the body would prepare itself to take flight and provides us with the energy needed to run. This would use up our Vitamin B reserve, making us feel tired, even exhausted.

The same thing happens with emotional stress. Several research studies have demonstrated that people who go through periods of intense work load or who suffer the loss of a loved one end up losing their Vitamin B reserve as well, showing symptoms of irritability, depression, and lack of energy.

Consuming a good quantity of dark green vegetables can help us prevent the consequences of stress.

Some vegetables also contain soluble fibers that clean arterial cholesterol. Soluble fibers ferment and change the contents of fatty acids in the colon, forming short-chain fatty acids that help reduce cholesterol production by the liver. They also maintain blood sugar levels stable by improving glucose's metabolism when fermenting.

Foods with a high content of soluble fiber are cactus leaves, apples, bananas, and carrots.

3. Yellows: Carbohyrates

Some fruits, cereals and legumes contain carbs that provide us with energy, as well as vitamins and fiber.

Some fruits contain Vitamin C, one of the most popular vitamins because it was the first to be discovered. When the Spanish were crossing the Atlantic towards America, the long journey combined with the sailor's poor diet made them suffer a vitamin deficiency called scurvy, which presented itself with bleeding gums. Nevertheless, according to the Indies treatises, when reaching tropical islands and eating fruits sailors were cured.

Vitamin C was discovered to be in citric fruits like orange, grapefruit, lime, and pineapple, as well as in kiwi, guava, and strawberries by the scientist Linus Puling, who also discovered that this vitamin favors the forming of scar tissue and helps prevent infections.

Vitamin C also intervenes in collagen formation, a protein that keeps our skin's integrity. As years go by, collagen fibers deteriorate and the skin turns thin and flaccid. Eating fruits rich in Vitamin C helps recover skin elasticity and youth.

Glyconutrients

The human body has the ability to transform sugars, but it cannot produce them by itself, which is why it is essential to get them from our diet.

There are eight saccharides that are essential to the cells communication process. If we eat them in adequate quantities, glyconutrients can reactivate the immune system, reduce allergies, and prevent cancerous tumors.

Even more, glyconutrients reduce inflammation processes like arthritis and normalize cholesterol and triglyceride blood levels. They also help in repairing the gastric mucosa, preventing ulcers and colitis.

Some glyconutrients can be found in carrots, pears, radishes, apples, and grapefruits.

When fruit is eaten raw, whole, and unpeeled (preferably), it is a great fiber source to help slow carb absorption rates.

Cereals (such as rice, corn, or wheat) and their products (like pasta, cookies, tortillas, and bread) provide carbohydrates. Carbs from cereals are digested easily and reach the blood at great speed, therefore providing energy to muscle cells. Hence, dining pasta and bread is recommended to marathon runners one day before the race. This fills their muscles with enough glycogen to provide energy during the marathon. In contrast, if you want to lose weight, your aim would be to provide no carb fuel for muscles, so that it utilizes fat reserves instead. This is accomplished by slowing the rate at which carbs reach the blood.

Carbs found in legumes like beans, lentils, and peas are digested slowly because the proteins present slow their passage through the stomach.

Proteins from legumes are known as incomplete proteins because they lack an amino acid called methionine. Nevertheless, if legumes and cereals are combined, like when we eat peas and rice or beans and tortillas, the quality of the protein is improved.

Cereals are also rich in different kinds of Vitamin B, which are essential for the nervous system. Whole grains are rich in nutritious substances, but when grinded they tend to become rancid. This is why when making flour, wheat germ is removed, therefore losing more than 20 nutritious substances. As an example we can look at white wheat flour, which, compared to whole wheat grain, lacks 60% of calcium, 71% of phosphorus, and 73% of Vitamin E.

Most cakes, cookies, bread, and boxed cereals are made with this kind of refined flours, therefore lacking thiamine and all the Vitamin B complex. An abuse in the consumption of refined cereals will end up by showing symptoms of anxiety, irritability, and tiredness. In contrast, by eating whole grain cereals we provide our body with the nutrients it needs to maintain health.

As a natural protection, all cereals have a husk called bran. It is a fiber that gets mixed up with our bolus and improves evacuation.

An adequate consumption of bran is elemental in maintaining our body's health. Fiber regulates the absorption of lipids, carbs, and proteins, and helps us prevent cardiovascular disease, cancer, hypertension, obesity, and diabetes.

Foods rich in insoluble fibers (like raw vegetables, fruits, whole cereals and legumes) facilitate intestinal evacuation.

Diverse health organizations recommend the consumption of 25 to 30 grams of fiber a day.

Examine the fiber content of your diet:

½ cup black beans	5 grams
½ cup lentils	4 grams
A medium apple	4 grams
A medium orange	3 grams
4 plums	3 grams
2/3 cup lentils	3 grams
A medium peach	2 grams
½ cup broccoli	2 grams

A medium banana	2 grams
½ cup of zucchini	1 gram
A slice of whole wheat bread	1 gram
½ cup of pasta	0.5 grams

Soy, a wonderful nutrient

In Asia, the soy bean has been considered both food and medicine for centuries. It is one of the five sacred crops, established so nearly five centuries ago by Shang-nung, a Chinese emperor.

Soy reduces cholesterol blood levels when they surpass 200 mg.

A research by Hamilton and Caroll studied the average cholesterol blood level in rabbits fed with soy's vegetable protein or with egg's animal protein. It revealed that the rabbits fed with eggs had cholesterol levels of 235 mg/dl, while those fed with soy protein had levels of 15 mg/dl.

In humans, research made by Anderson showed that soy proteins significantly reduce blood levels of total cholesterol, bad cholesterol (LDL), and triglycerides. DuPont reported to the FDA that, by eating 25 grams of soy a day, cholesterol levels may be reduced, preventing the risks of suffering cardiovascular disease.

Even more, soy has been demonstrated to be useful in reducing menopause symptoms like hot flashes and night sweats because of its isoflavone content, a substance that acts as natural estrogen.

However, eating high doses of soy may produce allergy. Therefore, it is important that those who consume high quantities of soy are attentive to perceiving any changes in their body. Allergy may be manifested as gastrointestinal problems, breathing difficulty, or skin rash.

After analyzing the low incidence of illness in Asian countries compared to American countries, Doctor Campbell recommends soy consumption, especially to people with high cholesterol and women with a high risk of breast cancer, reproductive organs cancer, or osteoporosis, as well as to those who suffer menopause symptoms and do not wish to receive hormonal treatment.

4. Blues: Fats

In the last few years, fats have become the diet tyrant. It has been said that fat is to blame for obesity problems and for most diseases. Nevertheless, recent studies report a whole different picture.

After evaluating 350,000 people, a study reported in the New England Journal of Medicine that it had been demonstrated that the amount of fat in a diet was not as important as the *type* of fat consumed.

Not all fats are bad and there exist some that actually produce health benefits.

Fats transport liposoluble vitamins like A, D, E, and K, form hormones, and maintain the body's temperature. They also protect internal organs like the heart and lungs, and act as insulation against the weather or against blows.

When reducing fat consumption under normal levels, a deficiency in hormone production is noted. This has been proved in anorexic women that, after submitting to very strict diets, stop menstruating for months or even years.

There are 3 types of fats:

1)   Animal Fats

2)   Marine Fats

3)   Vegetable Fats

1. Animal Fats

Among them you can find butter, bacon, lard, and cream. They contain a high percentage of cholesterol, a type of fat that adheres to arteries and forms a plaque that swells with time until it prevents adequate blood flow.

We may compare our arteries to freeways in which different vehicles flow: some trucks deposit bricks in the freeway, while others pick them up and take them to where houses are built.

Something similar happens in our arteries. Some substances, called low density lipoproteins (LDL), deposit cholesterol in the arteries, while others, high density lipoproteins (HDL), pick it up and take it to cells to produce hormones.

As new born babies, we used to have a good fat equilibrium, but as years go by and as we abuse the consumption of animal products, we increase the proportion of LDL, also known as bad cholesterol. This causes more deposits of cholesterol in our arteries than can be picked up, which ends up preventing blood flow. In the long run, this situation may cause a heart attack.

Another risk caused by eating animal or saturated fats is an increase in insulin production. By increasing the amount of saturated fat you eat, sugar will have a harder time getting through to muscles, turning muscles into insulin-resistant tissue: sugar cannot pass into the muscle and is in turn stored as fat. The body will then have to produce more insulin to try to get this sugar through, creating a vicious cycle.

2. Marine Fats

A study was made among the Eskimo population to estimate cholesterol blood levels. Before the study, scientists speculated that this population would show very high levels of blood cholesterol because their main diet consists of bear and seal fats. They were all surprised to find that most of them showed normal cholesterol levels.

After some studies regarding their diets, it was discovered that cold water fish, which were also a component of their diet, contain a fatty acid called Omega-3. This fatty acid increases the production of high density lipoproteins (HDL), which pick up cholesterol from the arteries and take it to hormone producing cells.

Omega-3 is mainly found in cold water fish like salmon, tuna, mackerel, herring, trout, and sardine. Other important sources of Omega-3 are canola oil and linseed seeds.

On the whole, the American diet is quite high on Omega-6 fatty acids, found in vegetable oils, and very low on Omega-3 fatty acids, found in cold water fish. Without an adequate intake of Omega-3, brain cells cannot form neurotransmitters, emit signals, and absorb enough serotonin to keep us relaxed and in a good mood.

A lack of equilibrium between Omega-6 and Omega-3 fatty acids has been associated with the appearance of chronic diseases such as diabetes, rheumatoid arthritis, colitis, depression, and cardiovascular disease.

To regain fatty acid equilibrium, begin by adding a tablespoon of linseed seeds to your daily diet. You can add it to your morning shake or combine it with the salad dressing. You can also find sufficient quantities of Omega-3 in canola oil and sunflower seeds. After several months of consuming more cold water fish, linseed seeds, and canola oil, you will begin to notice more resistant hair and nails, and find yourself to have a better mood every day.

3. Vegetable Fats

Vegetable fats can be found in seeds like pecans, almonds, pistachios, peanuts, and dried pumpkin seeds, as well as in different types of oils like corn, sunflower, sesame, and safflower oil, among others.

In the last 30 years, Americans have increased their consumption of polyunsaturated oils and margarines, which represents serious risks for their health.

In January 12, 1988, the American Medical Association reported in its internal medicine archives that a study had evaluated 61,471 women with a diet rich in polyunsaturated fats. This increased their risk of developing breast cancer by 69%. Another study in Iowa reported a 50% increase in cancer as a consequence of margarine and polyunsaturated fat consumption.

Western diets have over 20 times more omega 6 than omega 3 type fats, when a healthy ratio would be 4 to 1.

The most harmful fats in a diet are hydrogenated fats known as *trans fats*. These fats have been transformed by a hydrogenation process: vegetable lard, margarine, and mayonnaise.

Check labels and avoid consuming any product with hydrogenated fats: mayonnaise, snacks, potato chips, wheat flour tortillas, cookies, biscuits, pastries, etc.

Good Vegetable Fats

The fat founding seeds is very good for our health. Eat more pecans, almonds, pistachios, peanuts, pumpkin seeds, sesame seeds, and sunflower seeds.

Pecans Prevent Cancer

A recent report, published by the American Cancer Institute and by the International Cancer Research Foundation, showed that pecans contain great quantities of bioactive ingredients that strengthen human health. Among them are phytochemicals, vitamins, minerals, and fiber.

Numerous studies in lab mice demonstrate that pecans can prevent colon cancer and the proliferation of prostate and lung cancer cells. In these *in vivo* experiments, two specific phytochemicals, quercetin and kaempherol, have proved their efficiency in the fight against cancer.

The Benefits of Olive Oil

A study published by the American Journal of Nutrition reveals that women who consume oil and vinegar with their daily salad reduce their risk of a heart attack.

Olive oil contains a big quantity of alfa linoleic acid, a polyunsaturated fat that prevents the formation of plaques inside arteries. It is also possible that natural antioxidants contained in olive oil help stop LDL's oxidation (bad cholesterol's oxidation), the main cause of artery obstruction.

The *National Cancer Institute* reported on its *Journal* that a serving of olive oil a day reduces the risk of breast cancer by 25%. Women that live in Mediterranean areas, who follow diets rich in olive oil, have 50% less risk of developing breast cancer than American women do.

The most recommended olive oil is the extra virgin one, which has been pressed cold and has no chemical solvents.

It is best consumed cold. Avoid using it for frying since heating it saturates it quickly. The best oil for cooking is canola oil, rich in omega 3 and with a higher saturation temperature than olive oil.

A Fat-Rich Diet can be Beneficial to your Health

A recent study published by the *Neurology* journal, revealed that diet fats and proteins can protect against a type of dementia in people who have suffered a heart attack. This study showed that people who chose to follow a diet high in fats and low in carbs had 57% less chances of developing dementia after a heart attack, in comparison to those who chose to follow the traditional diet high in carbs and low in fats and proteins.

When eating a low-fat, high-carb diet (especially refined sugars and carbs), the body produces one of the most unhealthy saturated fats called palmitic acid, which reflects in high triglyceride levels in the blood.

In contrast, proteins and good fats help restore the walls of brain veins and arteries, while the Vitamin E contained in fats acts by preventing the oxidation of blood cholesterol.

Fat Myths and Truths

Myth: *The fats we eat are related to the amount of fat accumulated in our body.*

Not necessarily. We may consume little fat and nevertheless have a high percentage of body fat.

Some *light* foods are low in fat content, but contain starch. If we eat too many sugars or starch, we end up converting them to fats that are indeed deposited in our adipose tissue.

Three macronutrients provide calories. Carbs provide 4 kilocalories per gram; proteins provide 4 kilocalories per gram; fats provide 9 kilocalories per gram and, therefore, lowering their consumption is recommended. Nevertheless, fat consumption in the right amount is excellent to lose weight in a healthy way. In fact, fats help us lose weight and maintain our skin firm and lubricated.

Truth is that excessive fat consumption is not the only factor to blame when being overweight. If we eat more calories than our body needs, be it carbs, proteins or fats, we will accumulate them in our body.

Let's think of calories as the energy a steam train needs to reach its destination in a day. If we provide more coal than is necessary it will not burn and will just lie there, getting in the way.

People who cook with no fat and eat roast meat and salads sprinkled only with a little lime abound, also add many carbs to their diets, which end up turning into body fat.

Truth: *Eat fat and lose weight.*

Fats favor the release of a hormone called cholecystokinin, which notifies the brain of satiety. This way, adding a little   fat   to   each food may help eliminate appetite. Choosing healthy fats like almonds, peanuts, pecans, avocado, olive oil, and canola oil is recommended.

A recent study by Dr. Cummings in Washington University reported high blood levels of a hormone called ghrelin in people who had undergone weight loss diets.

It is believed that ghrelin production sends signals of hunger to the body as a survival measure. Ghrelin production increased 50% in those persons submitted to a weight loss diet, causing them to eat again and preventing them to keep a desired weight.

Ghrelin was found to be produced in some stomach cells, and its levels increased when the stomach was empty.

A diet moderated in fat can be the solution to keep us thin, for fats stimulate the release of enterogasterone, a substance that acts to inhibit secretion and gastric motility, slowing the release of fats towards the duodenum. As a result, when eating some fat, a fraction of what we ate remains in the stomach up to four hours or more, causing a feeling of satiety.

Myth: *Fat consumption increases blood triglycerides.*

Some of the people who undergo lab tests and show high triglyceride levels, immediately think they are related to the fats they eat. Nonetheless, an increase in triglycerides is generally due to carb abuse, such as high consumption of bread, tortillas, cookies, pastries, and sodas.

Truth: *Fats help us prevent premature aging.*

Vegetable fats are rich in Vitamin E, a very powerful antioxidant that slows skin aging and helps us prevent diseases related to cell deterioration like cancer, cataracts, pulmonary emphysema, arthritis, and Alzheimer disease.

Myth and Truth: *Vegetable fats are good, animal fats are bad.*

Hydrogenated vegetable fats, like margarine and vegetable lard, favor internal cholesterol production. Hence, they should be avoided.

In general, vegetable fats do not affect cholesterol blood levels.

Animal fats like butter, bacon, and cream, as well as sausages and some seafood like oysters and clams, increase blood cholesterol levels and favor the risk of cardiovascular disease.

In contrast, fats from seeds like almonds, pecans, and sesame, are sources of calcium, zinc, and vitamins that help improve our health.

It is key to recognize the importance that lies in changing our diet habits and reducing the intake of sausages like salami, wieners, and Spanish chorizo, which impoverish our health and put us at risk of suffering countless diseases.

Four Ways to Reduce the Amount of Fats Used while Cooking

1. Progressively reduce the amount of oil indicated in the recipe until you end up using half of the original amount.

2. When picking out canned tuna, prefer the one that comes in water.

3. Choose fresh cheeses over mature ones.

4. Reduce the amount of oil used to fry foods: cover the frying pan to keep humidity in and prevent food from sticking to the pan without the need to use more oil.

"Getting yourself used to the flavor of low fat foods requires 8 to 10 weeks," says Dr. Richard Mattes, nutrition professor at Purdue University. "But once used to it, we actually begin preferring these foods."

Change saturated fats for good fats

It is better to eat	Instead of
Semi skim milk	Whole milk
Low fat yogurt	Cream
Cottage or fresh cheese	Cheddar or swiss cheese

Sorbets	Ice cream
Skinned chicken or turkey	Duck or quail
Tuna canned in water	Tuna canned in oil
Fish	Oyster or clams
Herbs, wine	Pork or lamb meat
Hot chili pepper salsas	Thick sauces
Raw vegetables	French fries or pork cracklings
Water or tea	Milk shakes or chocolate milk
Natural popcorn	Buttered popcorn
Whole wheat bread	Sweet breads and pastries
Fruitcake	Cheesecake
Gelatin	Custards of puddings

We may sometimes not believe that in order to maintain our health we need nothing more than a simple and natural diet based on fresh vegetables and fruits, proteins, whole cereals, oils, and seeds.

Thanks to food, the opportunity of living a full life, both physically and mentally, is within our reach.

V

The Risks of a Bad Diet, moderation is the Key

The Risks of Excess Salt

Some experts state that eating too much salt could lower or even prevent the absorption of calcium in our body. When taken in excess, salt may over stimulate the adrenal glands, causing tiredness, chronic fatigue, and hypertension. Abuse in salt consumption increases our body's retention of liquids, adding an extra pressure to the heart. Finally, it creates a state of gastric acidity, establishing an ideal condition for developing ulcers. Eating salty foods has been related to acne, as well.

Lower Your Salt Consumption

To avoid salt abuse, limit your consumption of canned foods. To season your food, use a moderate amount of salt, dehydrated vegetables, or spices, and avoid the use of **chicken broth, soy sauce, and other seasoning sauces**. Likewise, reduce the amount of deli meats and sausages you eat.

Consuming a high amount of salt may cause accumulation of liquids within the body, reflected as swollen hands and feet. Water retention or persistent edema may be an indicator of cardiovascular disease, liver, bladder, or kidney problems, as well as the result of an allergy.

To reduce or prevent water retention, drinking two to three liters of water a day is recommended. Cranberry juice and hibiscus iced tea are recommended because of their diuretic effect, as well as green tea to which, when boiling, you can add some parsley or corn hairs.

In most populations, the amount of sodium intake supersedes the amount recommended to meet physiological needs. Even though mechanisms that regulate the clearance of excess sodium exist, this excess has been shown to be potentially harmful.

Several countries, as well as the World Health Organization (WHO), have adopted recommendations to reduce the intake of diet sodium, which must be between 2 and 4 grams a day, equivalent to 5 to 10 grams of sodium chloride (salt). Nowadays, American diet guides recommend a maximum of 2.5 g of salt, which is equivalent to half a teaspoon a day.

The relation that exists between high salt consumption and high blood pressure is the main reason for recommending a decrease in salt intake. There is solid evidence that an increase in the risk of developing cardiovascular disease is strictly linked with the sodium consumption rate. Even so, completely eliminating salt from your life is not advisable. The key is consuming it moderately.

The Risks of Alcohol

Recent studies have concluded that people who drink alcohol in small amounts have less risk of suffering cardiovascular diseases than people who do not do so. Nevertheless, those who drink excess alcohol lack this protective effect.

Even though our body's function when consuming alcohol has not been completely understood, it is known that consuming moderate quantities increases the levels of high density lipoproteins (HDL), commonly known as good cholesterol. Evidence confirms that alcohol lowers platelet aggregation, which in turn diminishes the risk of suffering a coronary artery obstruction.

In Mediterranean countries, where people drink one glass of red wine a day, the mortality rate for coronary disease has lowered. Even so, people who consume three or more glasses of alcohol a day have been observed to have heart muscle damage and other health problems.

Excessive alcohol consumption causes deficiencies of Vitamin B1, B2, and B6, niacin, folic acid, Vitamin C, magnesium, sodium, potassium, chlorine, and zinc.

Caffeine Addiction

Caffeine is an alkaloid that can be extracted from coffee, tea, or maté. According to Dr. John Hughes, psychiatry professor at Vermont University, caffeine is a substance that can create addiction and affect our emotions or actions at brain level, changing people's mood and conduct.

According to the definition proposed by the World Health Organization (WHO), an addiction is an intoxication state, periodic or chronic, produced by a substance's repeated consumption.

A cup of coffee can clear the mind and keep us alert and more concentrated. Nevertheless, coffee drank in excess can cause anxiety and tension.

Caffeine irritates the digestive lining and can cause heartburn; it has a diuretic effect and provokes decalcification of bones. It also reduces the body's Vitamin B concentration, affecting the health of the nervous system.

How to say goodbye to coffee?

Drinking great amounts of coffee affects our body's health. When deciding to abandon coffee, one or several of the following symptoms can be felt: fatigue, headache, depression, and a difficulty for concentration. This is owed to caffeine's addictive effects. However, it is worth the sacrifice, because these effects only last a few days and, by the end of a week, completely disappear.

Your health will benefit from reducing or stopping coffee consumption. Several studies coincide in that high doses of caffeine elevate the incidence of osteoporosis, ulcers, gastritis, tachycardia, and arterial hypertension. Other studies have demonstrated the relation that exists between people who consume higher quantities of caffeine and the presentation of abortion and fertility problems.

The latest studies indicate that some derivatives of caffeine stimulate insulin production. Therefore, if we abuse black coffee or cola drinks (even the diet ones) we would be in fact increasing our body's need of sugar, which would heighten our crave for sweets and, thus, our weight.

So how to eliminate or reduce coffee consumption? The best way to prevent withdrawal symptoms is to begin by gradually reducing the amount of caffeine consumed daily. If you drink five cups of coffee, four cups of tea, or six cans of cola drinks, you may begin by reducing your caffeine drinking 25% each week.

The first week begin by combining your favorite drink with a decaffeinated one in similar proportions. Or rather, when buying coffee beans, pick a blend made half of caffeinated and half of decaffeinated coffee.

Regarding cola drinks, begin by adding a little natural or mineral water, until the addiction completely disappears.

The Effects of Cola Drinks on Health

Drinking sugar sweetened sodas causes overweight problems and obesity. These drinks have alarming amounts of sucrose, glucose, and fructose. These are types of sugars reach the blood rapidly, cause an increase in insulin production, quickly get into tissues, and are turned into fat. Soda drinking and obesity have been related in up to 34% of cases.

It has been observed that drinking a liter a day causes a weight gain of about 2 lb every three weeks. Furthermore, drinking sodas displaces the consumption of other nutritious foods like fruits. This affects the quality of our diets. Sodas also damage dental integrity, dissolving teeth enamel and causing decay and cavities.

In children, drinking sodas has been related to hyperactivity, and testimonies show that when decreasing sugars and sodas to 50%, behavior improves in 42% of the cases.

Carbonated sodas or cola drinks may also cause sleep disorders because they contain very high amounts of caffeine. During sleep, the growth hormone is stimulated. Thus, a deep and sound sleep may help a child grow adequately, and an adult form muscle.

Even more, sodas that have gas also contain phosphoric acid, making calcium absorption more difficult and increasing the risk of osteoporosis.

The Diet Soda Myth

Most sugarless diet soda drinks do contain caffeine, a substance that stimulates insulin production. As previously stated, an insulin increase makes sugar blood levels lower and, hence, makes us feel hungry again in a few hours time. This way, people who drink big amounts of diet sodas will easily enter the "carb vicious cycle": eat and eat and eat.

Sugar Substitutes

Artificial sweeteners have been object of discussion for the last few years. In 1980, the World Health Organization accepted their use by virtue of its lack of apparent toxic effects.

However, consuming artificial sweeteners may have collateral effects in the body. When salivary glands detect a sweet flavor, the body prepares itself for digesting carbohydrates. Since it will not find them, the body is disconcerted and nevertheless prepares itself for the moment when carbs will be consumed. This takes the body to produce excess insulin. Some studies have found excess insulin production in people who abuse artificial sweetener consumption. And insulin, as we have seen, favors the storage of carbs as fat in the body.

The best would be for us to learn to enjoy the taste of natural foods, and not promote the consumption and excessive liking of sweet things in our diet, be it food or drink. Drinking natural water or skim milk is much better than drinking artificially sweetened sodas. Let's not forget that, furthermore, phosphoric acid contained in gaseous sodas causes bone decalcification.

Fructose

Consuming fructose has great advantages, especially when compared to artificial sweeteners. Fructose is a natural sugar that does not deceive the body. It has a Glycemic Index of 20, besides, causing very little insulin liberation. Its density is the same as that of sugar, so you can use it for baking. Nevertheless, limiting its consumption is recommended in order to not introduce many sugars in the blood and elevate the triglyceride levels, a state that can cause obesity and diabetes.

Testimonies

I am so happy... I've lost 7 pounds!

Hello, Paty, and thanks for the advice.

You know... I've lost 7 pounds since buying your book. I hadn't realized it, but after a week of buying the book I started including more fruits and vegetables in my diet, cutting down on refined flours, and eliminating cereals and yoghurt. I also stopped eating whole-oats cookies and am avoiding light sodas. I used to drink a couple of cans of Coke Zero a day, and usually had a raspberry and cream cheese crepe at the movies, along with a cappuccino. I did that almost every Saturday. Well... I stopped doing it. I also started drinking sugarless oat-water to help with constipation and it so happens that by combining all the foods of your color groups I began to feel better. What a great surprise I had yesterday when, walking in a shopping mall with my husband, I stepped in one of those weight/height/pressure measuring machines to find I had finally lost weight! From constantly being around 154 lb, I blissfully found my weight to be 145 lb! I confirmed it back home and was delighted.

Thanks again. I promise you I'll make it. I fly tomorrow to Venezuela, and I know I'll keep losing weight because my goal now is to go back to being as thin as before.

Thank you!

Claudia R.

VI

The Color Star Diet

After a long time trying to cover a myriad of nutrition knowledge, the twenty first century has arrived. As so often happens with these things, the search for this knowledge has made us come to extremes when it comes to diet recommendations.

Certain doctors, headed by Dr. Atkins, have stood by diets high in animal fat, which damage the circulatory system. Others have based their diets on the nutritional pyramid, recommending lots of carbs and thus increasing obesity, diabetes, and triglyceride problems. Some others have emphasized the importance of a diet high in   protein, overloading the kidneys and overproducing uric acid.

So which diet allows us to lose weight and improve our health?

The Color Star Diet

The Color Star Diet is the base of equilibrium. It proposes an ideal combination of different nutrients to obtain adequate hormonal response and allow the body to lose weight while staying healthy.

The Color Star Diet is an original and complete nutritional system that will help you improve your quality of life and reach the weight you have long desired. It will help you lose fat without losing muscle; it will increase your concentration and physical performance.

The Color Star Diet is the result of 27 years of study and private practice. It offers an easy and accessible method to lose weight without excessive sacrifice. It is the ideal diet: it adapts to you, to your likings and preferences... to your lifestyle.

The Color Star Diet provides the necessary amount of proteins to repair your muscles and tissues without damaging your kidneys. It is rich in beneficial fats, seeds, and marine oils that will help cleanse your cholesterol, build hormones, and allow you to lose weight while maintaining your skin's youth and lushness. It is also rich in fibers, vitamins, minerals and fitonutrients to help prevent illnesses and preserve health.

Color Star ABC's: 3 Quick Steps to Begin the Color Star Diet

These 3 simple steps will set you up to begin your diet with a goal and a time frame in mind.

STEP 1

FIND YOUR IDEAL WEIGHT

The first step in improving your health is finding your *Ideal Weight* and designing a diet that will help you reach it. You can find your ideal weight by using the weight-height table below:

Height		Men		Women	
Feet & Inches	Meters	Kg	Lbs	Kg	Lbs
4' 7"	1.40	...	...	40 - 53	88 - 116
4' 9"	1.45	...	...	42 - 54	92 - 119
4' 11"	1.50	...	...	43 - 55	94 - 121
4' 11½"	1.52	...	...	44 - 56	97 - 123
5' ½"	1.54	...	...	44 - 57	97 - 125
5' 1"	1.56	...	...	45 - 58	99 - 128
5' 2"	1.58	51 -64	112 - 141	46 - 59	101 - 130
5' 2½"	1.60	52 - 65	114 - 143	48 - 61	105 - 134
5' 3½"	1.62	53 - 66	116 - 145	49 - 62	108 - 136
5' 4½"	1.64	54 - 67	119 - 147	50 - 64	110 - 141
5' 5"	1.66	55 - 69	121 - 152	51 - 65	112 - 143
5' 6"	1.68	56 - 71	123 - 156	52 - 66	114 - 145
5' 6½"	1.70	58 - 73	127 - 161	53 - 67	117 - 147
5' 7½"	1.72	59 - 74	130 - 163	55 - 69	121 - 152
5' 8½"	1.74	60 - 75	132 - 165	56 - 70	123 - 154
5' 9"	1.76	62 - 77	136 - 169	58 - 72	128 - 158
5' 10"	1.78	64 - 79	141 - 174	59 - 74	130 - 163
5' 10½"	1.80	65 - 80	143 - 176	...	...
5' 11½"	1.82	66 - 82	145 - 180	...	...
6' 0"	1.84	67 - 84	147 - 185	...	...
6' 1"	1.86	69 - 86	152 - 189	...	...
6' 2"	1.88	71 - 88	156 - 194	...	...
6' 2½"	1.90	73 - 90	161 - 198	...	...
6' 3½"	1.92	75 - 93	165 - 205	...	...

A person with a narrow bones ought to aim for an ideal weight at the lower end of the range. A person of the same height but with wider bones could quite satisfactorily weigh in at the top of the range.

Medium-sized bones would land you on the middle weight range.

How to Determine Your Bone Frame Type

If in doubt, determine your bone frame type by measuring your wrist and comparing it to your height like this:

Your height in meters / Your wrist's circumference = Bone Frame Type

Results for Women

>11............□Narrow bones

10.1 - 11.. Medium bones

<11 ....Wide bones

Results for Men

>10.4..........Narrow bones

9.6 – 10.4...Medium bones

<9.6............Wide bones

If you find yourself to be a bit off your ideal weight by 4 to 6 pounds, don't worry. A slight variation in ideal weight exists, so you can stay like that. No one knows what your ideal weight should be better than you: that weight in which you have felt great, with energy and with good mental and physical performance.

It is important to highlight that the ideal weight you found through this table is only an approximate, for someone's ideal weight varies according to their muscle and body fat percentage. Some people exercise a lot and, because muscles weight more than fat, they may find themselves above their ideal weight without lacking perfect physical conditions. Others may be around their ideal weight yet have a high body fat percentage.

Muscle takes up the space of about a pound of ham, while fat represents a pound of lard. Therefore, if your measurements are not adequate, you may begin burning fat and substituting it with muscle today. Do not worry if you are not losing weight. You can be leaner while maintaining or even increasing your weight. The important thing is to *reduce your size*. This will be the best indicator of results.

STEP 2

FIND YOUR NUMBER OF COLOR STARS PER DAY

Once you know your ideal weight, and especially if you are above it, you need to find the amount of color stars you need to lose weight. How do you calculate your color stars?

Calculating your Color Stars per Day (for weight loss)				
Women´s Height	**Color Stars**		**Men´s Height**	**Color Stars**
< 4' 11"	3.5		< 5' 4½"	4
4' 11½" – 5' 6"	4		5' 5" – 5' 10"	5
> 5' 6½"	5		> 5' 10½"	6

A color star is a package that contains:

- 1 yellow (carb)
- 1 red (protein)
- 1 blue (fat)
- Unlimited greens

If you are a tall man who needs 6 color stars a day to lose weight, you can divide them like this:

Breakfast: 2 color stars = 2 carb portions, 2 protein portions, and 2 fat portions

Lunch: 2 color stars = 2 carb portions, 2 protein portions, and 2 fat portions

Dinner: 2 color stars = 2 carb portions, 2 protein portions, and 2 fat portions

Total = 6 color stars a day

- If you exercise aerobically:

Eat an extra carb (**yellow**) for every hour of exercise, and try to eat it *before* you exercise.

- If your exercise focuses on resistance (like lifting weights):

Eat a carb (**yellow**) and a protein portion, preferably *after* exercise.

An ideal way to accelerate your metabolism is to eat every three hours: you can eat half a fruit carb (**yellow**) in mid-morning and mid-afternoon. You can eat the fruit by itself since it has a slow Glycemic Index that does not affect insulin levels.

Remember there is a minimum of 3.5 color stars for women and 4 color stars for men. Ideally, eat every 3 hours to accelerate your metabolism.

STEP 3

FIND YOUR WEIGHT LOSS PERIOD

With the Color Star Diet, you will lose between 9 and 11 pounds every month.

That means you will lose a size every month.

A healthy weight loss time frame must be established in order for the diet to really work: lose weight safely, accelerate your metabolism, maintain firm skin, and not get the weight back.

EASY CALCULATION OF YOUR WEIGHT LOSS PERIOD

Present weight – ideal weight = _____ lb to lose

WOMEN: Pounds to lose ÷ 8 = _____ months (Weight loss period in months)

MEN: Pounds to lose ÷ 11 = _____ months (Weight loss period in months)

Note: Men have more muscle than women; this helps them lose weight faster.

Once you know the number of color stars to eat, you can begin designing your diet in the next chapter or, if you would like a more precise calculation, you can get one on www.dietadelosasteriscos.com.

Start Your Diet

If you happen to have some extra pounds, you are surely producing more insulin than is necessary. In order to lose weight, the first step to follow is to block insulin overproduction.

Insulin production may increase:

1. By eating more sugar than the body needs.

2. By consuming foods that take sugar to the blood very rapidly.

Our body has two organs that require sugar or glucose in order to function adequately: muscles and the brain.

When you want to lose weight, you should decrease the amount of carbs you eat so that you fuel the brain and only the brain... making muscles use stored fat reserves as fuel.

When you wish to maintain your weight, carbs must be eaten so that both the brain and the muscles are fueled, and when wishing to gain weight, an excess in carbs must be eaten so that the extra get stored as fat.

Protein portions remain stable and only increase when someone does resistance exercises like weight lifting, or during certain stages of life like childhood, adolescence, pregnancy, and breast-feeding.

Some diets or nutritional bars, like the Zone or Balance, recommend a fixed portion of carbs, proteins, and fats (40%, 30%, 30%) without adapting to each person's individual needs.

When someone consumes 30% of proteins in a maintenance diet or to put on weight, the kidneys may suffer damage.

In the Color Star Diet the amount of proteins remains the same when wishing to maintain weight or to lose it. Lowering protein intake is not recommended when wishing to lose weight because you need it to form muscles and to keep tissues firm.

On the other hand, carbs are the key when trying to lose or gain weight.

YELLOWS: CARBOHYRATES

It is important to eat carbs (*yellow*) in every meal to provide the brain with its sugar needs. The brain needs glucose to function. If it can't find it, it uses muscular amino acids as its source of energy. Consequently, a meal without carbs (*yellows*) causes muscle loss, while a meal that satisfies the brain's sugar needs allows the person to feel energized and begin burning fat reserves.

When muscles lack carbs (*yellows*), they use fat reserves as a fuel source. Thus, the ideal diet to lose weight would be one that satisfies the brain's needs but not the muscle's, obliging the latter to begin burning stored fat.

Sticking to a balanced diet when overweight is impossible, since the body itself lacks balance (it has too much stored fat and is producing more insulin than is necessary). To lose weight, carb ingestion (*yellow*) must be reduced and insulin overproduction blocked so that the muscles can finish burning stored fat. Once this happens, and the ideal weight is reached, carb quantities can be increased to satisfy both brain and muscle needs, maintaining an adequate balance.

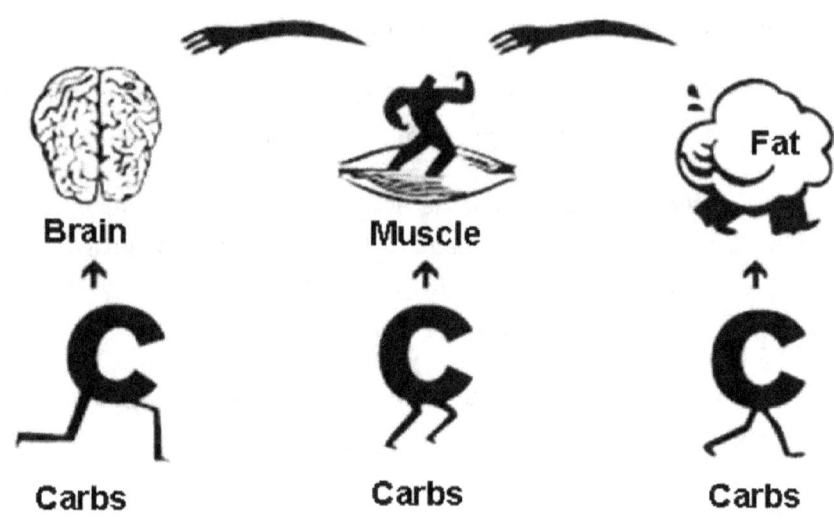

Design Your Own Diet

Once you know the number of color stars you need per day for your Weight Loss Period, you can begin designing your diet. Remember that each Color Star is a bundle that includes carbs (**yellows**), proteins (**reds**), and fats (**blues**). Greens are free to eat whenever you like to.

In order to keep your brain productive and alert, it is important to eat a carb serving (**yellow**) during every meal. Examples of a carb serving are 1 grapefruit, 2 cups of melon, 4 plums, or 1 pear. You may divide them throughout the day like this:

4 yellows a day may be distributed 1 per meal, 1⁄2 in mid-morning and 1⁄2 in the mid-afternoon:

1 yellow	Breakfast: 1 grapefruit
½ yellow	Mid-morning snack: 2 plums
1 yellow	Lunch: 2 cups of cantaloupe
½ yellow	Mid-afternoon snack: 10 grapes
1 yellow	Dinner: 1 pear

Remember that the first one to use carbs is the brain. Muscles use them if, and only if, the brain has leftovers. What we have to do then, to burn stored fat, is to make sure we only cover the brain's carb needs with 1 *yellow*, so that muscles use stored fat as energy when not finding leftover carbs.

Never eat all your daily *yellows* together during the same meal because too much sugar would reach the blood and end up stored as fat. To cover your brain's needs and to make your muscles use stored fat, pick one *yellow* per meal.

Where can carbs (*yellows*) be found?

Mainly, carbs can be found in fruits and cereals. A great difference exists between the two, though. While sugar from fruits, called fructose, reaches the blood slowly, starches from cereals reach it at great speed.

You can compare the energy carbs provide with fire: food represents the material that burns.

Think of a bonfire. Cereals are like newspaper: it burns immediately but is quickly consumed. Fruit, on the other hand, provides an energy that can be compared to firewood: it begins burning slowly, yet lasts a long time.

The brain needs a certain amount of carbs or sugars to work for four hours. By eating 2 cups of cantaloupe, 15 grams of sugar are gradually been taken into the blood and the brain takes what it needs. Little by little, more sugar reaches the blood... this covers the brain's needs for up to four hours. If, on the other hand, you eat a slice of bread, 15 grams of sugar reach the blood in a rush. The brain takes up what it needs ant the rest passes to muscles, preventing any fat burning from their part and hunger strikes again soon.

In order to slow down the process of carbs reaching the blood it is important that you combine food groups to form a color star. Sugars from cereals can be kept from reaching the blood stream too quickly by combining them with fiber, fats and proteins. This will make cereal sugars reach the blood at a slower pace and will keep your brain satisfied. When eating bread, combine it with some cheese; when eating cookies, eat some nuts or almonds as well.

Fruit and yogurt, on the other hand, do not need to be combined, even though they are *yellows*. You can eat them alone as a snack because their carbs have a Low Glycemic Index, and reach the blood quite slowly.

YELLOW PORTIONS (CARBS)	
It´s better to eat	*Than to eat*
(Low Glycemic Index)	(High Glycemic Index)
Tortoise Carbs	Hare Carbs
1 grapefruit (whole)	½ cup of rice
2 cups of cantaloupe	½ cup of pasta
2 oranges	1 slice of whole wheat bread
2 tangerines	2 corn tortillas
4 plums	4 whole grain crackers
1 apple	1 oatmeal cookie
½ cup of strawberries	2 cups of popcorn
1 pear	½ bread roll
2 peaches	4 teaspoons marmalade or jelly

These are only some *yellows* (carbs) as examples to help you design your menus. Full lists are available at the end of this chapter and in the back flap of this book.

Example for Distributing Yellows

Someone who needs 4 *yellows* (carbs) a day can distribute them like this:

Breakfast	Mid-morning snack	Lunch	Mid-afternoon snack	Dinner
(1 yellow)	(½ yellow)	(1 yellow)	(½ yellow)	(1 yellow)
1 grapefruit	½ apple	2 tortillas	2 plums	1 slice of bread

Pick a serving per meal to make sure you cover the brain's needs, maintain your muscle, and prevent a craving for sweets.

The Case with Men

Because men have a higher muscle proportion, and since muscles use glucose as fuel, men need a bigger amount of carbs.

A man with 5 *yellows* (carbs) per day may divide it like this: One for breakfast, 1 for a mid-morning snack, 1 for lunch, 1 for a mid-afternoon snack, and 1 for dinner. For example:

Breakfast	Mid-morning snack	Lunch	Mid-afternoon snack	Dinner
(1 yellow)	(1 yellow)	(1 yellow)	(1 yellow)	(1 yellow)
1 pear	4 plums	½ cup of rice	1 apple	2 corn tortillas

Recommendations

Carbs give energy to the brain and muscles. It is necessary, then, to consume them in order to maintain concentration and memory in optimal condition. When not eating *yellows* (carbs), the brain has no energy to function and we begin to suffer mental exhaustion or headaches.

On the other hand, by eating excess carbs, insulin production is stimulated and fat storage favored. Once fats are stored, sugar blood levels decrease, making us feel tired, dizzy, or sleepy.

To reach your goal, you must reduce the amount of carbs you eat. During the first three days, it is possible to feel anxiety for sweets, but gradually that need will diminish and be substituted by a peaceful feeling of well-being.

If you do not eat carbs or sugars on any given meal, your brain will feel the need for them. You will get a crave for something sweet, an anxiety that may be difficult to control. Or, even worse, you may feel lethargic and without energy.

Ideally, begin your diet by choosing your best source for *yellows* (carbs). By always picking at least one *yellow* (carb) serving per meal, you will allow sugar to feed your brain and maintain your good mood.

Fruits

If your lifestyle allows you to, choose fruit *yellows* during your first two weeks, and begin including cereals and other High Glycemic Index foods slowly.

Preferably, pick fruits that contain a lot of fiber and that have a Low Glycemic Index. The best options are cantaloupe, grapefruit, plums, and strawberries, although apples, tangerines, oranges, watermelon, papaya, and pineapple can also serve this purpose. Avoid fruits that have a High Glycemic Index like bananas or mango.

If you'd rather have fruit juice, add a little fiber to it so that the sugar absorption rate is slowed. You can also blend grapefruit juice with cactus pads (*nopales*) or celery.

BLUES: FATS

Fats are essential for forming hormones and to maintain your body's temperature. They help transport vitamins A, D, E, and K to such a degree that if fat consumption is stopped, a vitamin deficiency will present itself.

Yellows should be served with **a blue-fat portion during every meal**.

If you need *4 color stars*, eat **4 portions of fat**.

If you need *5 color stars*, eat **5 portions of fat**.

To maintain your health in optimal conditions, pick beneficial fats that help intestinal evacuation, reduce cholesterol blood levels, improve hormonal functioning, and keep your skin looking young and lubricated.

It is important to eat fats in every meal because fats stimulate Cholecystokinin production, a substance that sends satiety signals to the brain. Fats also form hormones, so that if people do not consume enough fats they may suffer from precocious menopause or andropause.

FAT SERVINGS:

1 teaspoon olive oil

1 teaspoon canola oil

2 teaspoons avocado

6 pecans

6 almonds

2 teaspoons ground linseeds

2 teaspoons sunflower seeds

1 1⁄2 teaspoons peanut butter

EXAMPLE, 4 COLOR STARS:

Breakfast	Lunch	Dinner
(1)	(1)	(2)
6 almonds	2 teaspoons avocado	2 teaspoons avocado
		1 teaspoon oil

EXAMPLE, 5 COLOR STARS:

Breakfast	Lunch	Dinner
(1)	(2)	(2)
6 Pecans	2 teaspoons avocado	2 teaspoons avocado
	1 teaspoon oil	1 teaspoon oil

As you can see, you don't have to worry about eating meat that's fried in a teaspoon of canola oil, or about a salad dressed in olive oil and vinegar.

REDS: PROTEINS

Protein consumption is essential in order to keep muscles and tissues healthy. When a diet lacks proteins, muscle is lost. This gains weight in the long run because each kilogram of muscle burns 45 calories a day, and, by not burning them, the body's metabolism slows and fat is accumulated.

When choosing reds (proteins), go for healthy choices.

- Eat only 4 eggs per week. When eating cheese, make sure it is low on animal fat. Prefer cottage, ricotta and mozzarella cheeses, or those that are fresh and low-fat.
- Eat low-fat and low-sodium hams like turkey or York ham.
- If you eat red meat, eat it only twice a week. Pick lean cuts like steaks or filets.
- Skin your chicken: the skin is full of saturated fats.
- Increase your fish consumption, especially cold-water fish like trout, salmon, tuna, sardines, mackerel, and herring, which contain Omega-3 to help you reduce blood cholesterol and benefit brain health.

PROTEIN PORTIONS (1 RED)

2 eggs

2 slices of ham

2 oz of meat

2 chicken thighs or legs

1 can of tuna fish (in water)

1/2 cup cottage cheese

2/3 cup low-fat cottage cheese

2 oz of fish

Eat 1 red for each *yellow* (carb). If you need 4 color stars a day, eat 4 reds:

Breakfast	Lunch	Dinner
(1)	(2)	(1)
2 oz low-fat Swiss cheese	1 can of tuna	4 oz of meat

Men have more body muscle percentage and thus eat more protein. If you are a man or a tall women who needs 5 color stars a day, eat 5 reds:

Breakfast	Lunch	Dinner
(1)	(2)	(2)
2 slices of ham	½ cup low-fat cottage cheese	2 oz of fish

GREENS: FREE FOODS

You can freely eat any amount of A-Vegetables which you can find in a list at the end of this chapter or in this book's back flap. These vegetables have very little carbs and don't affect insulin production. Preferably, eat them raw, increasing your vitamin and fiber consumption.

You can also use them to prepare stocks or vegetable soups, which will help you feel satisfied. Between meals, you can eat cucumbers or tomatoes with lime and chili powder or salt.

Your *yellows* (carbs) are your guide to choosing the amounts of everything else. For each *yellow* pick 1 red and 1 blue. Greens are free.

When eating at parties or reunions, make sure you never overeat any *yellows*. Counting fat and proteins can prove to be very difficult, but by taking care of the amount of carbs you eat, you'll notice important results in your weight loss.

EXAMPLE MENU: 4 COLOR STARS

Ideally, you should eat every three hours, including snacks for mid-morning and mid-afternoon.

Breakfast	1 grapefruit (yellow)
	3.5 oz. fresh grilled cheese with tomato sauce (red)
	1 teaspoon canola oil (blue)
Mid-morning Snack	½ big apple or 1 small one (½ yellow)
Lunch	1 tablespoon of mayonnaise (blue)
	1 can of tuna (red)
	Lettuce and tomato salad (green-free)
	4 whole grain crackers (yellow)
Mid-Afternoon Snack	2 plums (½ yellow)
Dinner	Vegetable salad with vinaigrette (blue)
	4 oz. chicken, beef or fish (2 reds)
	Cook it with vegetables and a teaspoon of oil (blue)
	Vegetable soup (with fat removed from broth or stock) (green-free
	1 ½ cup strawberries (yellow)

EXAMPLE MENU: 5 COLOR STARS

Breakfast	2 cups of cantaloupe (yellow) ½ cup cottage cheese (red) 6 almonds (blue)
Mid-morning Snack	1 pear or 1 yogurt (yellow)
Lunch	2 corn tortillas (yellow) 4 oz. chicken (2 reds) 4 teaspoons avocado (2 blue)
Mid-Afternoon Snack	1 apple (yellow)
Dinner	Free vegetable soup 4 oz. beef, chicken or fish stewed with vegetables (2 reds) Fried vegetables (1 blue) Vegetable salad with vinaigrette (1 blue) ½ cup of rice (yellow)

I recommend you to begin eating cereals once your diet's first two weeks have passed.

Choose fruit over cereals every chance you get. In a 3.5-color-star diet, for example, try to eat 2.5 *yellows* from fruit and only 1 from cereals. If your diet has 4 color stars, you can eat 2 and 2.

This diet will help you lose 11 pounds of fat per month.

If you begin to feel like you are losing weight at a slower rate, go back to fruit *yellows*, and preferably choose grapefruit, strawberries, and cantaloupe.

Some foods provide an important amount of both carbs and proteins, like legumes, yogurt, and milk.

Half a cup of beans has 12 grams of carbs and 7 grams of protein. Since they contain more carbs (*yellow*) than proteins (red), and to simplify your diet and its design, we will count these foods as *yellows* for menu purposes.

YELLOW SERVINGS (CARBS)

Fruits

Apples: 1 piece

Applesauce, unsweetened: 1/2 cup

Apricots, dried: 8 halves

Apricots, fresh: 4 pieces

Banana: 1/2 piece

Berries - Mixed: 1 cup

Berries - Blackberries: 1 cup

Berries - Blueberries: 3/4 cup

Berries - Raspberries: 1 cup

Berries - Strawberries: 1 ½ cups

Cherries: 1 cup or about 1 dozen

Dates: 2 pieces

Figs, dried: 3 small

Figs, fresh: 2 pieces

Grapefruit: 1 piece

Grapes: 20 pieces

Guava: 3 small pieces

Kiwi: 1 large

Lime: 4 pieces

Mango: 1/2 piece or 1/2 cup diced

Melon - Cantaloupe, cubed: 2 cups

Melon - Cantaloupe, wedge: 1/4 small melon

Melon - Honeydew: 1 cup cubed

Melon - Mixed melon balls: 1 cup or about 8

Mixed fruit: 3/4 cup

Nectarines: 2 pieces

Orange, navel: 1 medium

Orange, Seville: 2 pieces

Papaya: 1 cup

Peach: 1 large or 2 small

Pear: 1 piece

Pineapple: 1/2 cup cubed or 2 rings

Plum: 4 medium ones

Pomegranate: 2 pieces

Prickly Pear (tuna): 1 piece

Prunes: 4 pieces

Raisins: 20 pieces

Tangerines: 2 small pieces

Watermelon: 11⁄4 cups cubed or 1 small wedge

Carb-Rich Vegetables:

Beet: 1 cup

Carrots, raw: 4 medium ones

Corn kernels: 1⁄2 cup

Corn on the cob: 1 piece

Potato chips, baked (not fried): 15 pieces

Potato, baby, red-skinned: 3

Potato, baked: 1⁄2 medium

Potato, mashed: 1⁄2 cup

Pumpkin, cooked: 11⁄2 cups

Rutabaga, cooked: 3⁄4 cup

Squash, winter, cooked: 1 cup

Sweet potato, baked: 1⁄2 large

Turnips, cooked: 1/3 cup

Legumes

Beans: 1/2 cup

Black bean vegetarian burger: 3 oz patty

Broad beans: 1/2 cup

Chickpeas: 1/2 cup

Garbanzos: 1/3 cup

Green beans: 1 cup

Lentils: 1/2 cup

Peas: 1/2 cup

Soy (hydrated and texturized): 1 ½ cups

Soybeans, green (edamame): ½ cup

Tofu: ½ cup

Cereals

Amaranth: 1/3 cup

Bagel, whole-grain: 1/2

Barley, cooked: 1/3 cup

Bread roll: 1/2 piece, best if hollowed out

Bread roll, whole-grain: 1 small

Bread, hamburger bun: 1/2 piece

Bread, hot dog bun: 1/2 piece

Bread, pita, whole grain: 1/2 piece (6-inch diameter)

Bread, rye: 1 slice

Bread, sourdough: 1 slice

Bread, white: 1 slice

Bread, whole grain: 1 slice

Bread, whole wheat: 1 slice

Breadsticks, crispy: 2 pieces (6-8 inches long)

Bulgur, cooked: 1/2 cup

Cereal, All-Bran®: 1/2 cup

Cereal, Special K®: 1/2 cup

Cereal, whole-grain: 1/2 cup

Cookies, whole oatmeal: 1 big piece

Cookies, whole oatmeal: 2 small pieces

Cornstarch: 2 tablespoons

Crackers - Animal: 6 pieces

Crackers - Cheese: 14 small

Crackers - Melba rounds: 6

Crackers - Salty: 3 pieces

Crackers - Snack: 20 bite size, 5 round

Crackers - Triple-rye: 1

Crackers - Whole wheat: 6 little squares

Crepes (unfilled): 2 pieces

Croutons: 1/2 cup

English muffin, whole-grain: 1/2

Flour, refined wheat: 2 tablespoons

Flour, whole wheat: 21/2 tablespoons

Granola: 1/3 cup

Grits, uncooked: 2 tablespoons

Kasha (buckwheat groats, cooked): 1/2 cup

Ketchup: 4 tablespoons

Muffin, any kind: 1/2 piece or one small

Oatmeal, cooked: 1/2 cup

Oatmeal, whole grain: 1/2 cup

Orzo, cooked: 1/4 cup

Pancake: 1, 4-inch diameter

Pasta, cooked: 1/2 cup

Pasta, whole-grain, cooked: 1/2 cup

Popcorn, microwave, low-fat: 2 cups

Pretzels, sticks: 30

Pretzels, twists: 3

Rice, brown: 1/2 cup

Rice, cooked: 1/2 cup

Rice, precooked: 1/2 cup

Rice, wild: 1/2 cup

Wheat, shredded: 1 biscuit or 1/2 cup spoon-sized

Tortillas, white corn: 1 piece

Tortillas, yellow corn: 2 pieces

Waffle: 1, 4-inch square

Diary

Ice cream: 1/2 cup

Milk - Lactose-free: 1 cup

Milk - Powdered: 1/3 cup

Milk - Skim, 1% or 2%: 1 cup

Milk - Soy: 1 1/2 cups

Yoghurt, light, fruit: 1/2 cup

Yoghurt, natural: 1/2 cup

Yogurt, fat-free, frozen: 1/2 cup

Yogurt, fat-free, reduced-calorie: 1 cup

Drinks and Juices

Apple juice: 1/3 cup

Beer, light: 2 (12 oz each)

Beer: 1 (12 oz)

Cranberry juice, reduced-calorie: 1 cup

Cranberry juice, regular: 1/2 cup

Grape juice: 1/3 cup

Grapefruit juice: 1/2 cup

Juice bar, frozen: 3 oz bar

Orange juice: 1/2 cup

Pineapple juice: 1/2 cup

Plum juice: 1/3 cup

Soda: 1/3 cup

Sweets

Honey: 3 teaspoons

Sugar: 3 teaspoons

Angel food cake: 1 small slice

Apple pie: 1/3 slice (0.8 oz)

Cranberry sauce: 3 tablespoons

Fruit spread: 1 1/2 tablespoons

Gelatin dessert: 1/2 cup

Gumdrops: 6 pieces

Icicle: 1 piece

Jelly or marmalade: 3 teaspoons

Maple syrup: 1 1⁄2 tablespoons

Sorbet: 1⁄2 cup

RED SERVINGS (PROTEINS)

Eggs and Cheese

Eggs, medium: 2

Eggs, large: 1

Egg substitute: 1⁄2 cup

Egg whites: 4 pieces

Cheese - Cheddar, low-fat: 2 oz

Cheese - Colby, low-fat, shredded: 1⁄2 cup

Cheese - Colby, low-fat: 2 oz

Cheese - Cottage, low-fat: 2⁄3 cup

Cheese - Cottage, regular: 1⁄2 cup

Cheese - Feta: 1/4 cup

Cheese - Mozzarella, part-skim, shredded: 1⁄3 cup

Cheese - Mozzarella, part-skim: 3 oz

Cheese - Panela (fresh Mexican cheese): 3.5 oz

Cheese - Parmesan, grated: 3 tablespoons

Cheese - Ricotta, part-skim: 1/3 cup

Cheese - Swiss, low-fat, shredded: 1/2 cup

Cheese - Swiss, low-fat: 2 oz

Beef, Pork, others

Beef, lean: 2 oz

Ham: 2 slices (2 oz)

Wieners: 2 pieces

Lamb, lean cuts with no fat: 2 oz

Pork, lean cuts with no fat: 2 oz

Veal: 2 oz

Venison: 3 oz

Poultry

Chicken, skinned: 2 oz (2 thighs, 2 legs or 1/2 breast)

Duck, breast: 3 oz

Pheasant: 3 oz

Turkey, skinned: 2 oz

Turkey breast: 2 slices (2 oz)

Turkey ham: 2 slices (2 oz)

Fish and Seafood

Clams, canned: 1/2 cup

Cod: 3 oz

Crab: 3 oz

Fish: 2 oz

Halibut: 3 oz

Salmon: 3 oz

Scallops: 3 oz

Seafood: 2 oz

Shrimp: 3 oz

Tuna, canned in water: 1 can

BLUE SERVINGS (FATS)

Avocado: 2 tablespoons or 1/8

Butter: 1 teaspoon

Cream - Half-and-half: 2 tablespoons

Cream - Heavy (whipping): 1 tablespoon liquid or 4 tablespoons whipped

Cream - Nondairy creamer: 2 tablespoons

Cream - Nondairy whipped topping: 1/2 cup

Cream - Sour, fat-free: 3 tablespoons

Cream - Sour: 11/2 tablespoons

Cream cheese - Fat-free: 3 tablespoons

Cream cheese - Regular: 1 tablespoon

Cream: 1 tablespoon

Dressing (oil and vinegar): 1 tablespoon

Mayonnaise - Fat-free: 2 tablespoons

Mayonnaise - Reduced-calorie: 1 tablespoon

Mayonnaise - Regular: 2 teaspoons

Nuts - Almonds: 6

Nuts - Cashews: 4 whole

Nuts - Peanuts: 14

Nuts - Pecans: 6

Nuts - Pine kernels: 2 teaspoons

Nuts - Pistachios: 10

Nuts - Walnuts: 4 halves

Oil - Linseed: 1 teaspoon

Oil - Canola: 1 teaspoon

Oil - Olive: 1 teaspoon

Oil - Sesame seed: 1 teaspoon

Olives: 6

Peanut butter: 1 1/2 teaspoons

Seeds - Dried pumpkin: 1 tablespoon

Seeds - Flaxseed, ground: 2 teaspoons

Seeds - Sesame: 11/2 tablespoons

Seeds - Sunflower: 1 tablespoon

Tartar sauce: 1 tablespoon

A-VEGETABLES (FREE)

Artichokes

Asparagus

Bean sprouts

Bell pepper

Broccoli

Brussels sprouts

Cabbage Cactus pads (*nopal*)

Cauliflower

Celery

Cherry or grape tomatoes

Chili peppers

Coriander

Cucumber

Eggplant

Green onions or scallions

Green tomatoes

Hearts of palm

Hot peppers

Kale

Leek

Lettuce

Mushrooms

Okra

Onion

Parsley

Peppers

Pumpkin blossoms

Purslane

Radish

Spinach

Squash, summer

Swiss chards

Tomatillo

Tomato

Water chestnuts

Watercress

Zucchini

OTHER FREE FOODS

Beverages (with sweeteners, not sugar)

Hibiscus iced tea

Lemonade

Tea - Green

Tea - Red

Water, natural

Water, sparkling

Condiments

Capers

Fine herbs

Mustard

Oregano

Pepper

Saffron

Thyme

Vinegar

Moderately

Powdered chicken stock

Salt

Soy sauce

Worcestershire sauce

Foods that belong to 2 or more groups

Brownie: 1 small piece (1 yellow, 1 blue)

Cake: 3 tablespoons (0.8 oz) (1 yellow, 1 blue)

Chocolate - Kisses: 3 pieces (1 yellow, 1 blue)

Chocolate - M&Ms: 1/2 standard-sized bag (1 yellow, 1 blue)

Cinnamon Roll: 1/3 piece (1 yellow, 1 blue)

Doughnut: 1/3 piece (1 yellow, 1 blue)

Ice Cream Bar: 1 medium (1 yellow, 1 blue)

Ice Cream: 1/2 cup (1 yellow, 1 blue)

Pastries: 1/2 piece (1 yellow, 1 blue)

EXAMPLE MENU FOR A SEDENTARY WOMAN WITH A 4-COLOR-STAR DIET

Note: *Yellow* foods (carbs) appear underlined because they are the key for control in the Color Star Diet.

Day 1

Breakfast	<u>1 grapefruit (yellow)</u> 1 slice of turkey ham with 1 egg (red) 1 teaspoon canola oil (blue)
Mid-morning Snack	<u>½ big apple or 1 small one (½ yellow)</u>
Lunch	<u>4 salty crackers (yellow)</u> 1 can of tuna fish in water (red) Lettuce and tomato salad (green-free) 1 tablespoon vinaigrette (blue)
Mid-Afternoon Snack	<u>½ apple (½ yellow)</u>
Dinner	Water-based soup of free vegetables (green) <u>½ cup of spaghetti (1 yellow)</u> 4 oz of meat, chicken or fish stewed with vegetables (2 reds) Vegetable salad with apple vinegar, iodized salt, pepper 1 teaspoon of olive oil (blue)

Day 2

Breakfast	2 cups of cantaloupe (yellow)
	½ cup cottage cheese (red)
	6 pecans or almonds (blue)
Mid-morning Snack	2 plums (½ yellow)
Lunch	1 grapefruit (yellow)
	3.5 oz. Mozzarella cheese (red)
	Sliced tomato salad (green-free)
	1 teaspoon oil (blue), with oregano or basil
Mid-Afternoon Snack	½ apple or 10 grapes (½ yellow)
Dinner	4 oz meat stewed with vegetables (2 reds)
	Vegetable salad with vinaigrette (1 blue)
	(1 teaspoon of olive oil, apple vinegar, salt and pepper)
	1 ½ cup strawberries (1 yellow)

Day 3

Breakfast	1 cup of papaya (yellow)
	2 egg omelet fried with tomato, onion, peppers and mushrooms (red)
	1 teaspoon canola or linseed oil (blue)

Mid-morning Snack	10 grapes (½ yellow)
Lunch	1 slice whole grain toast (yellow)
	2 oz cubed chicken breast (red)
	2 teaspoons avocado (blue)
	Tomato and onion salsa
Mid-Afternoon Snack	2 plums or 1 tangerine (½ yellow)
Dinner	½ cup of rice (1 yellow)
	4 oz meat, chicken or fish stewed with vegetables (2 reds)
	Vegetable salad with vinaigrette (1 blue)
	(1 teaspoon of olive oil, apple vinegar, salt and pepper)
	Diet Jell-O

Day 4

Breakfast	2 cups of cantaloupe (yellow)
	Ham and cheese rolls: 1 ham slice and ¼ cup shredded Colby cheese (red)
	2 teaspoons avocado (blue)
Mid-morning Snack	1 orange (½ yellow)
Lunch	1 slice of whole wheat bread (yellow)
	1 slice of ham and ¼ cup shredded Colby

	cheese (red)
	Sliced tomato salad (green-free)
	2 teaspoons avocado (blue)
Mid-Afternoon Snack	<u>10 grapes or 1 orange or 1 cup of cantaloupe (½ yellow)</u>
Dinner	Vegetable soup
	<u>2 corn tortillas (1 yellow)</u>
	Seasoned, fried mushrooms topped with 3 tablespoons parmesan cheese (red)
	Tomato sauce with 1 teaspoon corn oil (1 blue)
	Vegetable salad and vinaigrette with 1 teaspoon olive oil (blue)

Day 5

Breakfast	<u>1 cup of cantaloupe (½ yellow)</u>
	<u>1 slice of toast (½ yellow)</u>
	1 egg, sunny side up, and 1 slice of ham (red)
	1 teaspoon canola oil (blue)
Mid-morning Snack	<u>1 small peach (½ yellow)</u>
Lunch	<u>2 corn tortillas (yellow)</u>
	3.5 oz. panela cheese (red)

	2 teaspoons avocado (blue)
	Free vegetable salad
Mid-Afternoon Snack	<u>1 cup of cantaloupe or 1 guava or 1 tangerine (½ yellow)</u>
Dinner	Vegetable soup
	4 oz. of salmon or 2 tuna cans (in water) (2 reds) fried with free vegetables
	<u>1 pear (yellow)</u>

Day 6

Breakfast	<u>1 yogurt (yellow)</u>
	½ cup cottage cheese (red)
	6 pecans or almonds (blue)
Mid-morning Snack	<u>½ pear (½ yellow)</u>
Lunch	<u>½ bread roll, hollowed out, or 1 slice of bread (yellow)</u>
	1 slice of ham and ¼ cup shredded Colby cheese (red)
	2 teaspoons avocado (blue)
Mid-Afternoon Snack	<u>½ apple or 2 plums (½ yellow)</u>
Dinner	Vegetable soup
	<u>½ cup of beans or lentils (yellow)</u>

4 oz. of stewed chicken (2 reds)

Vegetable salad with 1 teaspoon of olive oil (blue)

Diet Jell-O

Day 7

Breakfast	<u>1 grapefruit (yellow)</u> 1 egg omelet with mushrooms, peppers, and ¼ cup shredded, low-fat Colby cheese (red) 1 teaspoon canola oil (blue)
Mid-morning Snack	<u>1 can V-8 or tomato juice (½ yellow)</u>
Lunch	<u>1 slice toast(yellow)</u> 1 can of tuna fish in water (red) 1 tablespoon mayonnaise (blue) Cucumber and tomato salad
Mid-Afternoon Snack	<u>10 grapes (½ yellow)</u>
Dinner	Vegetable soup or broth 4 oz. hamburger patty (2 reds) <u>½ hamburger bun (or choose either the top or bottom part) (yellow)</u> Italian salad with vinaigrette (blue)

If you wish for a personalized diet according to your likings and life style, you can order it at www.dietadelosasteriscos.com

EXAMPLE MENU FOR A MAN WITH A 5-COLOR-STAR DIET

Day 1

Breakfast	<u>1 grapefruit (yellow)</u> 1 slice of turkey ham with 1 egg (red) 1 teaspoon canola oil (blue)
Lunch	<u>4 salty crackers (yellow)</u> 1 can of tuna fish in water (red) 2 tablespoons of mayonnaise (2 blue) <u>1 apple (yellow)</u>
Mid-Afternoon Snack	<u>2 cups of cantaloupe (yellow)</u>
Dinner	Soup of free vegetables in water (green) <u>½ bread roll (1 yellow)</u> 4 oz chicken stewed with vegetables (2 reds) 1 teaspoon canola oil (blue) Vegetable salad with 1 teaspoon of olive oil (blue)

Day 2

Breakfast	2 cups of cantaloupe (yellow) ½ cup cottage cheese (red) 2 teaspoons ground linseeds (blue)
Lunch	1 grapefruit (yellow) Sliced tomato salad 2/3 cup shredded mozzarella cheese (low-fat) (2 reds) 2 teaspoons of oil with oregano or basil (2 blues) 1 slice of whole wheat bread (yellow)
Mid-Afternoon Snack	1 ½ cups frozen strawberries (yellow)
Dinner	Chicken broth ½ cup spaghetti or rice (1 yellow) 4 oz. meat (2 reds) Cook it with vegetables and a teaspoon of oil (blue) Vegetable salad with vinaigrette (1 teaspoon of olive oil, apple vinegar, salt and pepper - blue)

Day 3

Breakfast	1 cup of papaya (yellow)
	2 egg omelet fried with tomato, onion, peppers and mushrooms (red)
	1 teaspoon canola or linseed oil (blue)
Lunch	2 corn tortillas (yellow)
	4 oz cubed chicken breast (2 red)
	4 teaspoons avocado (2 blue)
	½ cup of beans (yellow)
Mid-Afternoon Snack	4 plums or 2 tangerines (yellow)
Dinner	½ cup of rice (1 yellow)
	4 oz fish stewed with vegetables (2 reds)
	Cook it with vegetables and a teaspoon of oil (blue)
	Vegetable salad with vinaigrette (1 blue)
	(1 teaspoon of olive oil, apple vinegar, salt and pepper)
	Diet Jell-O

Day 4

Breakfast	2 cups of cantaloupe (yellow)
	Ham and cheese rolls: 1 ham slice and ¼ cup

	shredded Colby cheese (red)
	2 teaspoons avocado (blue)
Lunch	2 slice of whole wheat bread (2 yellow)
	2 slices of ham and ¼ cup shredded Colby cheese (red)
	4 teaspoons avocado (blue)
Mid-Afternoon Snack	1 apple (yellow)
Dinner	Vegetable soup
	½ cup of rice (1 yellow)
	2 peppers stuffed with 200g panela cheese (2 red)
	Tomato salsa fried with a teaspoon of oil (1 blue)
	Vegetable salad and vinaigrette with 1 teaspoon olive oil (blue)

Day 5

Breakfast	1 cup of cantaloupe (½ yellow)
	1 slice of toast (½ yellow)
	2 scrambled eggs with tomato sauce, peppers and onions (red)
	1 teaspoon canola oil (blue)
Lunch	2 corn tortillas (yellow)

	2/3 cup shredded mozzarella cheese (low-fat) (2 red)
	4 teaspoons avocado (2 blue)
	Free vegetable salad
	½ cup of beans (yellow)
Mid-Afternoon Snack	1 pear or 4 plums (yellow)
Dinner	Free vegetables
	4 oz. of salmon or 2 tuna cans (in water) (2 reds) fried with free vegetables
	1 teaspoon oil (blue)
	Vegetable salad with 1 teaspoon olive oil (blue)
	4 salty crackers (yellow)

Day 6

Breakfast	1 yogurt (yellow)
	2 rolls of ham (red)
	2 teaspoons avocado (blue)
Lunch	½ bread roll, hollowed out, or 1 slice of bread (yellow)
	2 slices of ham and ¼ cup shredded Colby cheese (2 reds)
	2 tablespoons of mayonnaise or 4 teaspoons

	of avocado (blue)
	1 yogurt or 1 cup of milk (yellow)
Dinner	Vegetable soup
	½ cup of beans or lentils (yellow)
	4 oz. of stewed chicken (2 reds)
	Cook it with vegetables and a teaspoon canola oil (blue)
	Vegetable salad with vinaigrette (blue)
	1 apple (yellow)
	Diet Jell-O

Day 7

	1 grapefruit (yellow)
Breakfast	1 egg omelet with mushrooms, peppers, and ¼ cup shredded, low-fat Colby cheese (red)
	1 teaspoon canola oil (blue)
Lunch	1 slice toast (yellow)
	2 can of tuna fish in water (2 reds)
	Cucumber salad with lime and 2 teaspoons of olive oil (2 blues)
	½ cup of corn kernels (yellow)
Dinner	Vegetable soup or broth

4 oz. hamburger patty (2 reds)

Fried with a teaspoon of oil (blue)

<u>1 hamburger bun (yellow)</u>

Italian salad with vinaigrette (blue)

If you accomplish a good distribution of **yellows** among your breakfast, mid- morning snack, lunch, mid-afternoon snack, and dinner your metabolism will activate and you will lose weight quicker.

To receive a personalized diet according to your weight, height, and physical activity, visit www.dietadelosasteriscos.com.

Testimonies

Dr. Paty Rivera,

Good morning. I write to thank you for your books, The Color Star Diet and Eating Well, the Best Medicine. Thanks to them, my wife's life has been saved, as well as the whole familiy's, since the mother is the family's cornerstone.

She had literally stopped breathing at night, and she woke up choking. She vows she even died once. I took her to see specialists and they did tests. She even saw an internist. Then someone recommended your book. She read it many times until she was completely convinced, and thanks to her studies she has saved her life.

She lost 40 pounds and currently weighs 114 pounds. Her whole image changed. She loves herself more and feels surer of herself. She is 36 years old and has two children aged 9 and 5. People who don't know her ask her why she has not had any children and are surprised to find out she has two!

My wife is alive and happy because of your books. Thank you, thank you very much.

Oh! And her name is Sandra Eulalia. She recommends your book to anyone she meets with an overweight problem, or cholesterol or triglyceride issues. She gives them your book as a gift...I actually bought one yesterday because she was going to give it away.

Thanks to your knowledge, Paty Rivera, and to faith, constancy, and my wife's life example, I begin today my new lifestyle and my new diet style as recommended by The Color Star Diet. I need to lose 53 lb. Let's see how long it takes me.

Greetings, and God bless,

Sergio Javier García Zapata

VII

On with Your Diet!

It is important to take intelligent decisions every time you eat. This will not only help you lose some weight, but will also make you feel full of energy and health.

When beginning a weight loss regime, one normally loses weight quite fast during the first couple of weeks. Say four pounds or more. This weight loss generally reflects a loss of water. Afterwards, the body begins to get used to the new diet and weight loss becomes less. Don't get discouraged. You'll be losing less weight but still be burning fat. Each kilogram of fat you lose represents 11 sticks of butter. Hence, you'll lose a lot in measurements.

Don't weigh yourself everyday. You may get discouraged and therefore lose a great opportunity.

Measuring your waist and hips every two weeks and writing down your accomplishments will be much more motivating. After a month, you will see several centimeters vanish from your waist.

Take a tape measure, wrap it around your waist, navel-high, and jot down your measurement.

Afterwards, wrap it over the bones on your hips. Write down the measurements in a notebook. You can start working on it today. Make a list of all the things you eat, for it is important to get know your present habits. Don't skip anything... not even a couple of peanuts. This list will help you see where you have to begin.

Analyze your breakfasts and what you can take out of them. If you're drinking two cups of coffee with milk, reduce it to one. If you normally eat one doughnut, change it for an oatmeal cookie. This way you'll be eliminating a yellow.

Eat a piece of fruit every meal, preferably raw and unpeeled, like an apple or pear. In case of an orange or grapefruit eat it in segments.

Prepare two big plates of raw salad, one for lunch and one for dinner. Add a dressing made with a tablespoon of olive oil and vinegar, lemon, mustard, and spices.

During breakfast, pick an egg, fresh cheese, or turkey breast-based dish, cooked with vegetables like tomato and onion or cactus leaves.

Cut simple sugars from your diet, like those in sodas, cakes, candies, and honey. Limit your consumption of alcohol to three cups a week, and preferably pick white wine, red wine, whiskey, or vodka.

Get rid of creamy dressings, gravies, egg white batter for frying, breadcrumb coatings, and bittersweet sauces.

Drink two liters of water a day, preferably cold, because cold water increases your internal calorie consumption.

Reduce your salt, soy sauce, broth, and Worcestershire sauce consumption, for they only make you retain water. Substitute your old habits with new ones.

Instead of using:	Use:

Cream Cheese	Cottage, tofu, or ricotta cheese
Cream	Low fat, blended cottage cheese
Whole milk	Semi-skim milk
Whole egg	Egg whites
Sausages	Turkey breast or York ham
Heavy sauces	Concentrated vegetable juices
Greasy meat	Steak, filet, or lean meat
Tuna canned in oil	Tuna canned in water
Sweet buns	Pumpernickel rye bread
Salt	Dehydrated spices or vegetables
Butter or lard	Seed or vegetable oils
Manchego or Chihuahua cheese	Fresh cheeses
Breaded or fried fish	Ceviche, grilled fish
Shrimp or oysters	Salmon or herring
Potato or beet	Spinach, broccoli, or cauliflower

Some foods favor insulin production and, therefore, fat storage. You need to rid them from your diet if you wish to lose weight. Among them we can find refined sugar, bread made with refined wheat flour (the whiter the bread, the more insulin it produces), and potatoes (unpeeled potatoes produce less insulin than peeled potatoes do). Carrots, when raw, produce little insulin. When cooked, however, their carbs are chemically changed, causing an increase in insulin production. The longer a rice grain is, the less insulin it produces. Something similar happens with bananas: the greener they are, the less insulin they produce.

How to Begin

A good day may begin with a breakfast rich in fiber: one unpeeled apple or 2 cups of cantaloupe, 2 oranges in segments or a good papaya slice with cottage or fresh cheese, almonds or nuts.

Or you can eat a slice of rye bread or 1/2 a whole grain bagel, or 1 bran or oatmeal cookie alongside an omelet or fresh cheese cooked with vegetables.

Some patients ask me if it's Ok to skip meals. Several studies have demonstrated that what really matters is not *how much* you eat, but rather *what* you eat. Skipping breakfast has been proven to make you consume excess calories in your next meal. Nevertheless, what happens if you eat a breakfast rich in sugars? The problem is that those who eat a lot of carbs for breakfast as well as those who skip this meal will end up eating many more calories than they should during the rest of the day.

If you eat a lot of **carbs-yellows** in a single meal, you cause your sugar levels to rise abruptly. Since your brain cannot store that much sugar, and since it is dangerous for sugar to remain within the arteries (because it damages them), the pancreas produces insulin, making sugars pass into muscles where it is stored as fat. In this way, blood sugar levels decrease and you begin feeling hungry again.

The results from a study made in St. Luke Roosevelt Hospital Center in New York, where two types of breakfast and fasting itself were evaluated, are very interesting. Both obese people and people with ideal weight were selected to participate. One group received a 350 calorie breakfast based on whole grain oatmeal. A second group got a 350 calorie breakfast of sugared cornflakes, while the third group fasted, drinking only water. For the rest of the morning, those who had oatmeal felt less hungry by lunchtime and ate 30% less calories than those who had had sugared cornflakes for breakfast. What was really surprising was that those who ate cornflakes were so hungry that they consumed as many calories as those who had had only water.

The reduction in calorie consumption was especially significant on overweight people who had had oatmeal. What, then, is the difference between eating cornflakes and eating oatmeal? Both cereals are similar calorie-wise, but oatmeal has much more fiber. It seems that eating fiber acts as an appetite suppressor and reduces the speed with which sugar reaches the blood.

LUNCHTIME

There's nothing better than a salad for lunch. A mixture of green leaved vegetables with fresh cheese and basil, or with tuna and tomato, dressed with a good vinaigrette. You can choose two *tostadas* (dried corn tortillas), a slice of whole grain bread or a fruit serving for your yellow carbs.

When eating out: Order a salad to begin. Never order chorizo (highly-seasoned pork sausage), chistorra (fried spicy Spanish sausage), or French fries. Pick a vegetable soup or a good broth instead of a cream. As a main dish, eat lime chicken or grilled fish instead of breaded beef or lasagna.

DINNER

Begin your meal with a protein serving, stimulating the secretion of glucagon (a hormone that liberates sugar from the liver and sends it into the blood stream). By beginning with the main dish, you recover your blood sugar levels before having eaten too much.

Prepare your main dish based on chicken, meat, or fish, cooked with vegetables or wine and spices. Or rather, meat stew with tomato or fish in tomato sauce with broccoli and mushrooms. Avoid gravies and white sauces because they contain refined sugars. Three tablespoons of these sauces are equivalent to your yellow carb serving.

If you eat meat with tortillas, prefer corn ones instead of wheat ones, for the former have more fiber. Or rather, eat with a slice of whole grain bread.

Eat a good soup, preferably made of free vegetables or broth.

Studies made in England report that people who consume watery soups instead of creamy ones (like vegetable soup or broth), consume less calories per meal than those who skip the soup. Remember that you can also pick a serving of yellow carbs, like 1/2 cup of pasta or rice, though bean or lentil soup would be a better option because of its fiber contents.

Include a good raw salad during dinner, remembering that when vegetables are cooked they lose their fiber content. Eat crunchy vegetables to cause a feeling of satiety. Dress them with olive oil and vinegar or with a little of parmesan cheese and aromatic herbs.

At the end, have diet Jell-O or, if you still have a yellow, a good dessert based on seasonal fruits. Preferably, eat the fruits raw and unpeeled.

Try drinking a lot of water. It is vital for your health, and when you drink it cold your burn calories as well.

Regarding alcohol, do not drink more than two glasses per meal. Either have wine, vodka, or whisky, for they don't have any carbs, or use up your yellow carb with a beer or a glass of rum with diet soda.

RECOMMENDATIONS

If you really want to lose weight, you have to change your lifestyle and adopt a new healthier one. This will help you gain, not only good looks, but also health.

You may begin by eating slower in a time span no shorter than 20 minutes, because the quicker you eat the more you eat. When eating too quickly, the stomach has no time to signal the brain about its fullness, and you keep eating without realizing you are completely satisfied. Get used to leaving the fork in your plate between each bite. Avoid eating while watching TV or reading the newspaper. Sit down at the table with tranquility, conscious of what you are doing. A lot of people eat to diminish anxiety, anger, solitude, or boredom. Practice your favorite sport or take a walk instead.

Avoid having sweets and fattening food around.

Use small dishes.

Always go to the supermarket after eating. If you don't, your appetite will make you buy calorie-rich foods.

Eating between meals is OK when choosing well. An apple or half a grapefruit are light snacks that kill hunger.

It's better to eat a little five times a day than to eat two times in excess.

Munching on a celery stick or on a carrot piece when weak is a good option.

Do not include sugar, sweets, or sodas in your diet. Avoid fried foods and prepared snacks.

Prefer fish and chicken breast to beef and pork, as well as green and yellow vegetables to white ones (like potatoes).

Lower your bread and rice consumption and increase your fruit and vegetable one, for they provide fiber.

When chewing and absorbing cucumbers, raw carrots, or bran, energy and time are required, which is why a person with a high-fiber diet can feel satisfied without eating too much.

A high-fiber diet is bigger in volume and needs more chewing time, which produces greater quantities of both saliva and gastric juices. This additional liquid is mixed with food in the stomach, thickening the fiber. This distends the stomach and quickly gives a lasting feeling of satiety.

Fiber causes the small intestine to absorb calories slower, allowing you to eat more and keep losing weight.

As a general rule, eat at least three cups of vegetables a day. This will give you enough fiber to complete digestion and make you feel full.

Eating four to five times a day is recommended.

It is better to eat several light meals a day than one or two abundant ones, for it has been proven that people who eat several times a day burn more calories.

Sumo wrestlers, for example, fast for long periods and then eat an abundant meal once in order to lose muscle and gain fat.

When eating very heavy meals insulin blood levels are increased.

Eating five times a day, with four- to five-hour intervals in between, allows us to keep sugar blood levels stable, allowing better performance, concentration, and creativity.

Take Care of Your Skin

The speed at which we get older may accelerate or slow down according to our diet.

According to Doctor Cooper, obesity is an accelerating factor. By losing weight, quitting smoking, and exercising, you can significantly slow down the aging process in a very short time.

Skin is one of the indicators of aging. Skin is stretched with each weight gain. When your weight varies, stretch marks appear and the skin loses its ability to contract as it should, showing tissue flaccidity. This is why following a healthy regime is ideal, allowing us to lose weight slowly and not regain it.

An unbalanced diet may cause skin disorders. In contrast, a diet with enough zinc and Vitamin A can help give a healthy and youthful appearance. Zinc helps tissue repair and Vitamin A increases the cellular exchange rate and prevents skin dehydration. Good sources of zinc are beef, eggs, seafood, and green-leafed vegetables like watercress, Swiss chards, and spinach. You can find Vitamin A in carrots, watermelon, cantaloupe, peach, mango, broccoli, and red pepper.

Vitamin C improves the skin's circulation and helps collagen production, an essential protein for keeping tissues firm. Some foods rich in Vitamin C are chile, guava, grapefruit, orange, lime, pineapple, cabbage, and Brussels sprout.

Doctor Blumberg recommends drinking 6 to 8 glasses of water a day in order to keep tissues hydrated and regain a youthful aspect.

THE IMPORTANCE OF WATER

One of the best habits you can acquire is that of drinking 8 glasses of water a day. The human body is calculated to need 3 liters of water a day. One liter and a half, approximately, is obtained from solid foods like fruits and vegetables, which provide important quantities of water. The other liter and a half must be consumed by drinking.

Water is essential for life, for our cells' correct functioning. Drinking it in enough quantities helps us correct and prevent tiredness and weakness in general, constipation, high fever, intoxication, dehydration, and some liver and kidney problems.

Water and fiber are vital for intestinal evacuation. Not drinking enough water may cause constipation. This happens because if the water drunk is not enough, the body protects itself by absorbing it from the colon area, drying up feces and making it hard to evacuate.

When drinking herbal tea or hot water with the juice of half a lime during lunchtime, we favor fat clearance.

Imagine that you are about to wash a dish full of grease. You will need hot water for the fat to be dissolved. The same thing happens with food. Orientals, a population with a very low obesity index, drink green tea or jasmine tea.

If you wish to lose weight, you should avoid foods that produce a high amount of insulin and choose those that produce less. You may use the following list to help yourself pick these foods.

Avoid (high amounts of insulin):	Prefer (low amounts of insulin):
Baked potato	Beans
French fries	Lentils
Mashed potatoes	Peas
Short-grained rice	Long-grained rice
Instant rice	Precooked rice
Rice flour	Whole oats
Atole (Mexican hot maize drink)	Tomato juice

White bread	Rye bread, unsifted (pumpernickel bread)
Baguette or bread roll	Bran bread
Sweet potato	Raw or frozen vegetables
Honey	Low sugar marmalade
Cooked carrots	Raw carrots
Beet	Fresh fruits
Cornflakes	Apple in pieces
Popcorn	Zucchini
Pumpkin	Whole oats
Boxed cereals	Oatmeal or bran crackers
Refined cookies	Spaghetti *al dente*
Instant noodles	Cantaloupe
Banana	Unpeeled grapes
Raisins	

Your Friend the Cold

Cold is another useful factor to accelerate the weight loss process. Our body keeps itself at a temperature of 37°C.

Take advantage of a cloudy or cool day by not covering yourself too much: your body will burn calories in order to keep its temperature normal.

Testimonies

Hello,

My name is Laura and I'm very happy! I no longer feel fatigued, and it's wonderful to feel well after so many years of suffering it. You were right to tell me that with the Color Star Program I would get better.

Two weeks ago, when I went to see you, I weighed 132 pounds. I now weight 125, and still want to lose 4 more. I feel good. I want to exercise, walk or swim for 30 minutes a day.

I had started to feel overweight and uncomfortable. I was starting to wear blouses outside skirts and pants, feeling insecure... but now I feel great and happy.

As I mentioned, I spent my days at home, spiritless... not hungry but craving sweets. Now, little by little, I am retaking my activities: I've been out dancing, to the movies, to concert, and to restaurants. Last Sunday I was out for almost 12 hours, something I hadn't been able to do for over six years.

My husband is very surprised, and we are both quite happy. I carry on with my medical treatment, but I'm sure that by continuing this way, I'll be able to stop taking medicines. Thanks to God, my life has changed.

Second Letter

I feel better every day. A month ago, I had the pleasure of meeting you, and I've already lost 11 pounds. I now weight 121 pounds!

Chronic fatigue has vanished. It's wonderful, and I feel very happy, for I'm retaking the normal life I had six years ago. I can now spend 8 or 10 hours away from home, and I'll soon get back to work.

Laura Juárez

VIII

Lies that Hamper Your Weight Loss

In recent years, the concept of diet has been varying. For 18 years, we have been taught to be afraid of fats, and that is why we feel safe buying low-fat food products. Nevertheless, a lot of these products have extra carbs added (like cornstarch) to give them consistency, ending up as excess sugar or carbs stored as body fat.

1. SUGAR FREE COOKIES AND DIET CANDIES

These foods are sold with the label "sugar free", and we trust them, since they are made for diabetics. However, they contain other kinds of carbs that sabotage our weight loss attempts (like flour or cornstarch).

Some foods don't have any sucrose, commonly known as sugar. What they do have, though, is flour derivatives that elevate sugar blood levels and favor the production of the hunger hormone, insulin. Furthermore, an excess consumption of this type of sugars may cause diarrhea, cramps, and the desire to eat again.

2. LACTOSE-FREE AND/OR SOY MILK

Lactose-free milk is very good for people who cannot digest lactose, the natural sugar that milk contains. It has, though, other carb sources that may also elevate sugar blood levels. When drinking this milk, you may feel at peace, believing that you are avoiding calories, but many times this kind of milk has the same number of calories as common milk has, even if they come from different   sources.

You may drink a cup of this milk and count it as 1 yellow serving. Or, if you have no lactose problems, you can pick skimmed milk instead of whole milk, thus avoiding saturated fat consumption.

If you want to lose weight, follow the Diabetes Association recommendations: count how many carbs you eat to maintain your sugar blood levels stable and keep your body thin and healthy.

3. WHOLE GRAIN COOKIES OR BREAD

Many people think that any kind of whole grain cookies or bread help when losing weight because of their fiber content. But the truth is that almost all of them are made with refined flour with very little fiber (from 0 to 5 g). Furthermore, the type of bran added to them is so grinded that the carbs it contains practically reach the blood at the same time as with white bread.

Preferably, choose low fat cookies made with whole wheat, which have 2 g of fiber for each 15 g of cookie. As for bread, eat pumpernickel bread (unsifted rye bread).

4. GRANOLA BARS OR BOXED CEREALS

The nutrition pyramid recommendations gave as a result the birth of the cereal industry, which has stuffed supermarket shelves with granola bars and boxed cereals.

These products contain a great amount of carbs. Eaten with a glass of milk and some fruit, the body's sugar needs are surpassed.

Let's remember that counting carbs is very important in order to reach our ideal weight.

5. JUICES OR NATURAL FRUIT DRINKS

Each cup (240 ml) of these products has only 5% of natural juice. The rest is a mixture of water with artificial flavorings that sometimes may have up to 150 calories and a very significant carb amount (up to 2 to 3 yellows).

Instead of this product, I recommend you have whole fruit and a glass of water. If you want to drink juice, dilute it with water and add some kind of fiber like cactus leaves or bran.

6. CEREALS, GRANOLA, SEEDS, AND DEHYDRATED FRUIT MIX

We generally relate this kind of snack with health and well-being. Nevertheless, every 3 teaspoons provide 130 calories, so that if you eat the recommended serving, you'll be consuming 800 calories! In addition, some mixes contain grated coconut, an ingredient rich in saturated fat that elevates cholesterol blood levels.

If you wish to eat this mix as a snack, limit yourself to ¼ cup. It would be much better to eat an unpeeled apple, for example, or a cup of cantaloupe, or an orange in sections, snacks that leave you feeling much more satisfied.

7. LOW-FAT POTATO CHIPS

The phrase "Low-fat" makes it appear like whatever it is that you're eating will help you lose weight. The surprise is that since potato consumption became popular in Europe, the obesity index increased. This is owed to the great amount of starch contained in them, which reaches the blood at great speed and elevates sugar levels. When eating too many carbs, the potato ends up being stored as fat.

You have to take into account that the potato's preparation process affects the speed at which sugar reaches your blood. When eating boiled, unpeeled potatoes, the absorption speed is slower. In contrast, when eating baked or mashed potatoes, sugar is absorbed at great speeds and passed to the muscles, or ends up turning into fat.

8. DIET COLA DRINKS AND BLACK TEA

Caffeine consumption stimulates insulin production. By abusing these kind of products, sugar blood levels decrease and the desire to eat carbs arises. As a result, caffeine incites us to eat and eat. If you wish to lose weight, I recommend you substitute decaf coffee for black coffee, and lemonade or plain water for cola drinks, as well as lowering your chocolate and black tea consumption.

9. HONEY AND FRUIT JAMS

Most jams and marmalades are made with fruit bases and specific quantities of sugars or carbs. Corn syrups are generally added to marmalades. An ideal would be to read the labels, choose marmalades low on carbs, and eat the smallest amount possible.

10. CARROTS, BEETS, GREEN BEANS, AND CORN

Some people think they can eat these vegetables unlimitedly just because they are vegetables. Nonetheless, they have a greater amount of sugars and carbs than other vegetables and, therefore, we must limit our consumption.

In the case of carrots, eating them raw is recommended, for their fiber slows carb absorption speeds and gives a sate sensation. On the other hand, when eaten cooked, in soups, or as a side dish, their sugars may unfold into starch and reach the blood even faster.

11. MARGARINES OR BUTTER SUBSTITUTES

These products contain hydrogenated fats that increase cholesterol levels, and are therefore harmful to our health. It would be ideal to cook with vegetable fats like canola, linseed, or sunflower oil, and to use olive oil for salad preparation.

Limit your oil consumption to three to four teaspoons a day, but do not avoid it, for it contains essential fatty acids and Vitamins A, D, E, and K, which favor our organism's health.

Testimonies

Dr. Paty,

I write to congratulate you for sharing your knowledge. Your Color Star regime is a marvel.

I had been a vegetarian for 10 years. For health reasons, I had to stop eating soy, my only protein source along with legumes. I gained 16 pounds in the last few months, and I couldn't get rid of them.

I fasted, stopped eating all kinds of fat, ate little, exercised daily and still nothing. I visited a nutriologist and her regime made me feel worse. I was full of carbs and ate very little fruit. I began to think something was wrong with me, and I began stressing a lot. I felt tired, my hair began to fall out. I had to do something about my diet right away.

I started your diet as a way to include more proteins in my meals and I finally made it! It is incredible. I can eat all the food I like, especially fruits and vegetables, and now I eat fish, light cheeses and some egg as proteins. I still eat a little tofu because I like it so much, and I feel great. I still exercise and feel wonderful. I'm still losing weight, my pants fit again, and in a couple more weeks I'll begin my maintenance phase.

I was doubtful in the beginning, thinking it was just another diet. I was beginning to get used to the chubby me, trying to eat well... but no! This way of eating is a miracle!

Thank you. Thank you very much. May God continue to guide you and help us chubbies get healthier and feel better.

Greetings,

Karin Serralde

IX

Lose Those Extra Pounds While Having Fun!

We all wish to look and feel good without much sacrifice. Many times, we submit ourselves to a diet to lose weight and end up quitting it because we cannot follow such a strict regime. In the beginning, we feel full of willpower and are capable of taking a prepared dinner to a friend's house who has a party or has invited us over for dinner. But as time goes on, we get tired or get discouraged, and all the work it takes to follow the diet, as well as the fact that you get more and more isolated if you follow it, ends up making you throw away all your good intentions.

For many people, undertaking a diet means closing up at home and forgetting about enjoying life. It does not have to be this way: with some good choices you can learn to eat healthily and get rid of those extra pounds.

According to some statistics, 48% of adults feel that eating out is an essential part of their lifestyles. Restaurants and school cafeterias serve more than 50 billion meals a year. With a little knowledge of losing-weight principles, you can go out to have fun, try new things, and still lose weight.

TIPS FOR EATING OUT

To begin, order tomato juice, mineral water with lime, white wine, or red wine.

Pick only one carb serving. For example, if you order a beer, do not eat bread. Or if you wish half a dessert, do not drink beer nor order spaghetti, rice, tortillas, or bread.

Begin with your main dish. Select simply prepared foods. To eat with less fat prefer baked, boiled, grilled, or steamed dishes, as well as those cooked on their own juice. Avoid fried foods and those topped with cheese, cream, or sauce.

To prevent eating an excessive amount of carbs or sugars, order chicken, meat or fish with any vegetable, and avoid dishes prepared with potatoes, corn, beets, green beans, and cooked carrot.

You can pick a steak prepared in mixed fresh herbs, lime, or mustard; fish with a garlic and oil based sauce or tomato sauce; chicken in tomato sauce or grilled.

Avoid foods fried with eggs or breadcrumbs, as well as topping your food with gravies or sauces (like sweet-sour or barbecue sauce).

Remember to eat reasonably sized portions as well, for restaurants normally serve very big portions. Try to share your order with a friend, or ask to have the leftovers packed to take home. It is better to pay the whole meal and eat only half, than it is to store half a ration as body fat.

CAREFUL WITH SALADS!

According to the American Dietetic Association, a salad dish can contribute up to 1,000 calories because commercial dressings sometimes have plenty of starch. If you add croutons, cheese, and bacon bits on top of it, a result will be a calorie excess.

It is better to pick raw vegetables. They can be green leaves like lettuce, Swiss chard, spinach, or watercress, or rather tomato, red or green peppers, hearts of palm, or asparagus. Dress them yourself with vinegar and olive oil. You can add condiments or spices. If your salad has goat cheese or turkey ham, count it as your main dish. Afterwards, you may eat half a serving of dessert if you didn't have any bread.

The best desserts you can choose are fruit (*yellow*) or ice cream (½ cup for 1 *yellow*). You can also order a cappuccino without sugar or a third of a piece of cake, and count that as your carb.

Some more useful tips for eating out follow.

TACOS

Choose:

- 2 tortillas or 1 beer (1 *yellow*)
- Mineral water
- Beef or chicken (red), scallions, mushrooms, and some
- avocado (blue).

Make sure to choose lean meats like steak, filet, or shredded meat. The size of the meat serving must be equivalent to your palm's size without counting fingers. Avoid barbecued pork and very greasy meats, which contain very harmful animal fats, especially for your circulatory system.

Salsas prepared with tomato, hot chili peppers, and onions are free (greens). You can finish with sugarless mints.

SANDWICHES

Choose a simple filling:

- Ham, chicken, fresh cheese, or shredded meat
- Avoid sandwiches with fried fillings
- Eat only the top or bottom half of the bread (1 *yellow*)
- Order bottled or mineral water with lime

You can add a side dish of green salad or a broth.

HAMBURGERS

Eat only half the bun (the top or the bottom half) if your diet indicates only one *yellow* for that meal.

Order your hamburger without cheese and add only a little ketchup. As a side dish, you can have raw salad with lime or Italian vinaigrette, or rather, choose a hamburger with lettuce and tomato. Avoid hamburger combos that include French fries and soda (together they add up to 9 or 10 *yellows*, which is too much sugar for a single meal, and will all end up stored as fat).

Eat either six French fries, half the hamburger bun (the top or bottom part), or six chicken nuggets. If you do not like simple water, you can ask for sparkling water and add some lime.

ITALIAN RESTAURANTS

You can begin with *carpaccio* as an entrée or a tomato and mozzarella cheese salad.

When ordering pasta, order only ½ cup of pasta prepared with tomato, mushrooms, and cheese, or with tomato, peppers, and meat or seafood.

In case of ordering a pizza, eat only a slice and do not eat any more bread. Eat it with a good chicken salad or cheese with vinaigrette.

JAPANESE RESTAURANTS

Pick a non-fried sushi roll or half an order of Yakimeshi (fried rice with vegetables). You can follow with a teppanyaki (grilled chicken or shrimp with vegetables) or a cucumber and crab salad. Shrimp or chicken brochettes are a good option too.

CHINESE RESTAURANTS

Chinese food contains a vast amount of starch, so be very careful with it.

Avoid breaded and fried foods, as well as bittersweet sauce. The best dish to have would be a chop suey with half an order of rice.

INTERNATIONAL FOOD RESTAURANT

If you have the chance to pick where to go, this type of restaurant may be the best choice, for in it you will find a great variety of dishes to choose from. You can have a vegetable soup or dishes prepared with red or white wine.

Always ask the waiter how a dish is prepared, and avoid any recipe that contains flour or cornstarch. As an entrée, choose artichokes, mushrooms, asparagus or hearts of palm.

Pick a good salad and dress it with olive oil and vinegar. Avoid dressings such as Thousand island, Roquefort, and French (these are normally thickened with flour or cornstarch, of which 3 tablespoons make 1 *yellow*).

As a complement, you can drink a good cup of wine. Enjoy every bite and, above all, enjoy life, enjoy your friends, enjoy the conversation. A good friend as company can enrich you and fill that space that you cannot see, but that is always there, yearning to live.

Testimonies

After years of looking for the most appropriate diet for me, and with no results, I bought your book The Color Star Diet a few months ago asking myself... will this work?

I am now happy to follow the recommendations you give. I've lost a size in a month and a half. I eat deliciously and without worrying about taking a menu with me wherever I go, be it a restaurant or a friend's house. I spent lots of money on diets, limiting my buying other things. I now thank God for having met a person so honest and professional in her field of work.

May God bless you. Wholeheartedly,

Adriana Rodríguez Peña

www.ingramcontent.com/pod-product-compliance
Lightning Source LLC
Chambersburg PA
CBHW070032300526
45794CB00001B/458